T0261837

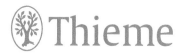

Neuro ICU Procedure Atlas

Jack I. Jallo, MD, PhD
Professor and Vice-Chair
Academic Services;
Director
Division of Neurotrauma and Critical Care
Department of Neurological Surgery
Sidney Kimmel Medical College
Thomas Jefferson University
Philadelphia, Pennsylvania, USA

David F. Slottje, MD
Neurosurgeon
Sentara Martha Jefferson Neurosciences
Charlottesville, Virginia, USA

108 illustrations

Thieme
New York • Stuttgart • Delhi • Rio de Janeiro

Library of Congress Cataloging-in-Publication Data is available from the publisher.

Important note: Medicine is an ever-changing science undergoing continual development. Research and clinical experience are continually expanding our knowledge, in particular our knowledge of proper treatment and drug therapy. Insofar as this book mentions any dosage or application, readers may rest assured that the authors, editors, and publishers have made every effort to ensure that such references are in accordance with **the state of knowledge at the time of production of the book.**

Nevertheless, this does not involve, imply, or express any guarantee or responsibility on the part of the publishers in respect to any dosage instructions and forms of applications stated in the book. **Every user is requested to examine carefully** the manufacturers' leaflets accompanying each drug and to check, if necessary in consultation with a physician or specialist, whether the dosage schedules mentioned therein or the contraindications stated by the manufacturers differ from the statements made in the present book. Such examination is particularly important with drugs that are either rarely used or have been newly released on the market. Every dosage schedule or every form of application used is entirely at the user's own risk and responsibility. The authors and publishers request every user to report to the publishers any discrepancies or inaccuracies noticed. If errors in this work are found after publication, errata will be posted at www.thieme.com on the product description page.

Some of the product names, patents, and registered designs referred to in this book are in fact registered trademarks or proprietary names even though specific reference to this fact is not always made in the text. Therefore, the appearance of a name without designation as proprietary is not to be construed as a representation by the publisher that it is in the public domain.

Thieme Medical Publishers, Inc.
333 Seventh Avenue, 18th Floor
New York, NY 10001, USA
www.thieme.com
+1 800 782 3488, customerservice@thieme.com

Cover design: Thieme Publishing Group
Typesetting by Thomson Digital, India

Printed in USA by King Printing
Company, Inc.   5 4 3 2 1

ISBN 978-1-68420-017-7

Also available as an e-book:
eISBN 978-1-68420-018-4

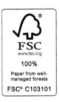

FSC
www.fsc.org
100%
Paper from well-managed forests
FSC® C103101

Contents

Contents

Contents

Contents

Contents

Contents

Preface

Dear Reader,

The concept of this book came about at one of our neurosurgical meetings when Tim Hiscock, the former executive editor at Thieme Publishers, commented on the lack of a basic procedure manual for the neurocritical care unit. My first thoughts were that this information is readily available in a variety of sources. However, after some discussion, it was agreed that a single resource would be beneficial to practitioners at the bedside. Many months later with inputs from our house staff, advanced practice providers, and authors, we developed the text you now hold. We hope that it is helpful to a clinician at the bedside and may serve as a resource.

The chapters are structured to be easily reviewed with a brief introduction, relevant anatomy, indications/contraindication, equipment needed, and technique as well as possible complications.

This work would not be possible without the time and effort of our authors and my thanks goes out to them. Additionally, the team at Thieme Publishers has been exceptional in seeing us through the process and if not for the tireless efforts of Ms. Snehil Sharma, we would not have completed this work in a timely fashion.

Jack I. Jallo, MD, PhD
David F. Slottje, MD

Contributors

Rachid Assina, MD, RPh
Assistant Professor
Department of Neurological Surgery
Rutgers New Jersey Medical School
Newark, New Jersey, USA

Amanda Carpenter, MD
Resident Physician (Neurosurgery)
Rutgers University
New Brunswick, New Jersey, USA

Celina Crisman, MD
Assistant Professor of Neurosurgery
University of Massachusetts
Department of Neurosurgery
Worcester, Massachusetts, USA

Michael Cohen, MD
Neurosurgeon
Eastern Maine Medical Center
Northern Light Health
Bangor, Maine USA

Amandeep S. Dolla, MBBS, MD
Clinical Assistant Professor
Department of Neurology/Division of
    Neurocritical Care
Sidney Kimmel Medical College
Thomas Jefferson University
Philadelphia, Pennsylvania, USA

Adam D. Fox, DPM, DO, FACS
Associate Professor of Surgery
Rutgers NJMS
Division of Trauma and Critical Care
Medical Director, JEMSTAR Air Medical
    Program
Newark, New Jersey, USA

Ira Goldstein, MD
Director
Center for Neurotrauma
Division of Neurosurgery at NBI
Rutgers New Jersey Medical School
Newark, New Jersey, USA

Robert F. Heary, MD
Professor of Neurological Surgery
Hackensack Meridian School of Medicine
Chief of Neurosurgery
Mountainside Medical Center
Montclair, New Jersey, USA

R. Nick Hernandez, MD
Neurosurgeon, NeuroScience & Spine
    Associates
Penn Medicine Lancaster General Health
Lancaster, Pennsylvania, USA

Yehuda Herschman, MD
Neurosurgeon
South Florida Neurosurgery
Atlantis, Florida, USA

M. Omar Iqbal, MD
Resident Neurosurgeon
Department of Neurosurgery
Rutgers University
Newark, New Jersey, USA

John Kauffmann, PA-C
Physician Assistant
Department of Neurosurgery
RWJBarnabas Health
New Brunswick, New Jersey, USA

Gurkirat Kohli, MD
Resident (Neurosurgery)
School of Medicine
University of Rochester Medical Center
Rochester, New York, USA

Brent Lewis, MD
Emergency Medicine Physician
Jersey City Medical Center
Jersey City, New Jersey, USA

John W. Liang, MD
Director
Neurosciences ICU
Mount Sinai West;
Assistant Professor
Departments of Neurosurgery & Neurology
Mount Sinai Health System
New York, New York, USA

Neil Majmundar, MD
Neurosurgery Resident
Department of Neurological Surgery
Rutgers New Jersey Medical School
Newark, New Jersey, USA

Ahmed M. Meleis, MD
Assistant Professor of Neurological Surgery
Department of Neurosurgery
Albany Medical Center
Albany, New York, USA

Matthew S. Parr, MD
Resident Physician
Department of Neurosurgery
School of Medicine
University of Alabama Medical Center
Birmingham, Alabama, USA

Nitesh V. Patel, MD
Department of Neurosurgery
RWJBarnabas Health
Rutgers University
New Brunswick, New Jersey, USA

Irene Say, MD
Resident Physician
Department of Neurosurgery
Rutgers University
Newark, New Jersey, USA

Amna Sheikh, MBBS, MD
Intensivist
Department of Critical Care
Winchester Medical Center
Winchester, Virgina, USA

David F. Slottje, MD
Neurosurgeon
Sentara Martha Jefferson Neurosciences
Charlottesville, Virginia, USA

Elena Solli, MD
Resident Physician in Neurosurgery
Rutgers New Jersey Medical School
New York, New York, USA

Matthew Vibbert, MD
Assistant Professor
Neurology and Neurological Surgery
Sidney Kimmel Medical College
Thomas Jefferson University
Philadelphia, Pennsylvania, USA

David A. Wyler, MD
Assistant Professor
Anesthesiology and Neurological Surgery
Director of Anesthesiology Neurocritical Care
Assistant Program Director
Anesthesiology Residency Program
Sidney Kimmel Medical College
Thomas Jefferson University
Philadelphia, Pennsylvania, USA

1 External Ventricular Drain

David F. Slottje, Nitesh V. Patel, and Ira Goldstein

Abstract
External ventricular drains (EVDs) are a common and useful tool in the Neuro-ICU. Here the following topics related to insertion of an EVD are discussed in detail: relevant anatomy and physiology, indications/contraindications, equipment, technique, complications, and expert suggestions.

Keywords: ventricular drain, external ventricular drain, ventriculostomy, cerebrospinal fluid, hydrocephalus, intracranial pressure

1.1 Introduction

An external ventricular drain (EVD) is a catheter, inserted via a cranial opening, through the dura and brain parenchyma, into the ventricular system. Cerebrospinal fluid (CSF) flows through the catheter into an external collection burette. The CSF column height in the catheter tubing reflects the intracranial pressure (ICP). Typically, a transducer is connected to the tubing to measure and record the ICP. The pressure is reported in cm H_2O or mm Hg. The tubing system contains a valve stopcock which can be occluded or opened to allow egress of CSF into the burette. When the stopcock is open, the height of the burette can be adjusted to regulate the flow of CSF. CSF will drain into the burette when the ICP exceeds the height of the burette (see ▶ Fig. 1.1).

1.2 Relevant Anatomy and Physiology

Cerebrospinal fluid is produced by the choroid plexus. Prominent tufts of choroid plexus are most commonly located in the atria of the lateral ventricles, within the third ventricle, and at the foramina of Monro and Luschka. CSF flows from the lateral ventricles, through the foramina of Monro, into the third ventricle, through the Sylvian aqueduct, into the fourth ventricle, through the foramina of Luschka and Magendie, and into the subarachnoid cisternal spaces around the brain, spinal cord, and spinal nerves. The CSF is resorbed from the subarachnoid space into the superior sagittal sinus via the arachnoid granulations (see ▶ Fig. 1.2).

In an adult, the central nervous system contains roughly 150 cc of CSF at any given time. Under normal conditions, the ventricles only contain 25 cc of CSF, with the remainder being located in the subarachnoid spaces. The majority of subarachnoid CSF lies within the lumbar cistern. The CSF is replaced roughly three times daily, with a typical adult generating 450 cc of CSF per day.

Imbalance of CSF cycling can be due to overproduction, or more commonly impeded resorption. Overproduction of CSF is encountered rarely in the setting

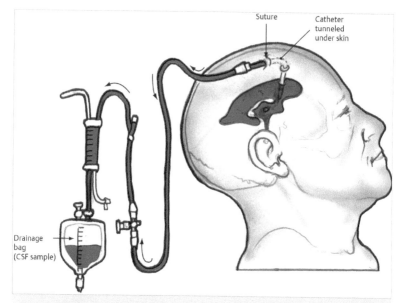

Fig. 1.1 Schematic of external ventricular drain (EVD). (Modified with permission from External Ventricular Drain and Ventricular Access Devices. In: Nader R, Gragnanielllo C, Berta S, et al, Hrsg. Neurosurgery Tricks of the Trade. Cranial. 1st Edition. Thieme; 2013.)

of choroid plexus papillomas. Disruption of CSF resorption can be classified as obstructive or nonobstructive.

Obstructive hydrocephalus results from any macroscopic blockage of CSF flow at any point in the CSF pathway. This may be due to a blood clot, tumor, other mass lesion, or cerebral edema. Common scenarios resulting in obstructive hydrocephalus include subarachnoid/ventricular hemorrhage obstructing the third ventricle or Sylvian aqueduct, posterior fossa lesions (i.e., tumors, intraparenchymal hemorrhages, cytotoxic edema from cerebellar stroke) obstructing the fourth ventricle, or intraventricular lesions such as a colloid cyst which may act as a "ball valve" intermittently obstructing the third ventricle (see ▶ Fig. 1.3).

Nonobstructive hydrocephalus results from congestion or scaring of the arachnoid granulations, preventing the resorption of CSF into the bloodstream (see ▶ Fig. 1.4). Nonobstructive hydrocephalus is commonly seen in the aftermath of bacterial meningitis or following subarachnoid hemorrhage. Less commonly, certain tumors, such as pineocytomas, may cause nonobstructive hydrocephalus by shedding large amounts of proteinaceous debris.

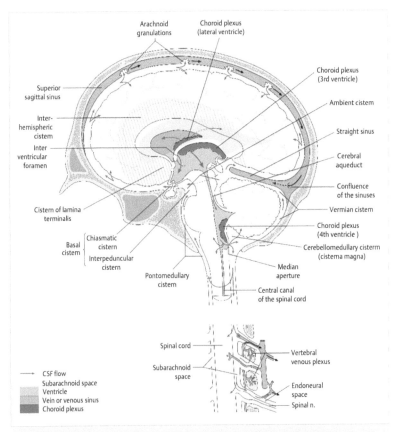

Fig. 1.2 Circulation of cerebrospinal fluid (CSF). (Reproduced from: Meyers S, Hrsg. Differential Diagnosis in Neuroimaging: Brain and Meninges. 1st Edition. Thieme; 2016.)

1.3 Indications

The indications for insertion of a ventricular drain fall into three broad categories—ICP monitoring, CSF diversion, and intrathecal access. In many disease states, the ventricular drain may serve multiple purposes concurrently.

1.3.1 ICP Monitoring

A ventricular drain allows for direct measurement of ICP by establishing a mobile fluid column in continuity with the CSF space. Measurement of the ICP may be desirable to direct therapy in patients with intracranial hypertension, to monitor

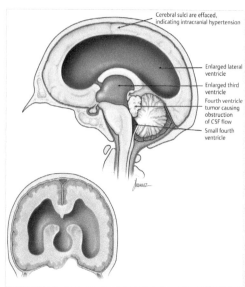

Fig. 1.3 Obstructive hydrocephalus due to tumor compressing cerebral aqueduct. (Reproduced from Hydrocephalus. In: Alberstone C, Benzel E, Najm I et al, Hrsg. Anatomic Basis of Neurologic Diagnosis. 1st Edition. Thieme; 2009. doi:10.1055/b-005–148822)

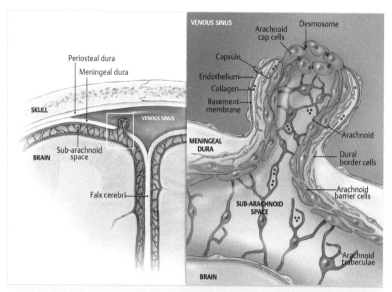

Fig. 1.4 Arachnoid granulations in superior sagittal sinus. (Reproduced from The Fine Structures of the Meninges. In: DeMonte F, McDermott M, Al-Mefty O, Hrsg. Al-Mefty's Meningiomas. 2nd Edition. Thieme; 2011.)

for the development of intracranial hypertension in comatose patients, or to diagnose various disease states when there is clinical suspicion for intracranial hypertension. Of note, when ICP monitoring is the only anticipated application for a ventricular drain, a fiber-optic ICP monitor may be preferred, given the lower risk of infection and less invasive nature of this procedure (see Chapter 5).

1.3.2 CSF Diversion

By allowing for external drainage of CSF, a ventricular drain can relieve build-up of CSF and reduce ICP. This function of a ventricular drain is especially useful and potentially life-saving in the setting of acute hydrocephalus. It may also be useful to afford modest ICP reduction in cases of global brain injury even with relatively normal CSF circulation. Additionally, CSF diversion can be used to clear the ventricular system of debris (i.e., blood or proteinacious material) that is anticipated to clog the arachnoid granulations and would otherwise result in hydrocephalus. Lastly, CSF diversion may be used to relieve pressure on a CSF fistula to prevent CSF leak and promote healing and closure of the fistula.

1.3.3 Intrathecal Access

A ventricular drain can be used to administer medications directly into the intrathecal space, or to obtain a sample of CSF for analysis. Ventricular drains are rarely placed primarily for intrathecal access, but they are frequently used for this purpose when placed for other indications.

1.4 Contraindications

The following are relative contraindications to insertion of a ventricular drain:
• Coagulopathy
• Thrombocytopenia
• Recent antiplatelet therapy
• Uremic platelet dysfunction
• Recent thrombolytic therapy
• Mass lesion obstructing catheter trajectory
• Scalp infection

1.4.1 Special Situations

Periventricular pyogenic abscesses pose significant risk during ventricular drain insertion given that rupture of such lesions through the ependyma may cause ventriculitis, rapid neurologic decline, and death. Similarly, the approach vector of a ventricular catheter should avoid peri- or intraventricular neurocysticercosis cysts as puncture of these lesions prior to steroid administration will generate a potentially fatal inflammatory response.

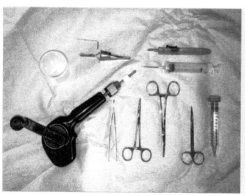

Fig. 1.5 Cranial access kit.

1.5 Equipment

The majority of equipment needed for ventricular drain insertion is contained in a pre-packaged cranial access kit (see ▶ Fig. 1.5). Below is a list of the necessary equipment:
- Ventriculostomy catheter, trochar
- Twist drill
- CSF collection system burette
- #15 or #10 blade scalpel
- Lidocaine with epinephrine
- Cap, mask, gown, sterile gloves (× 2), perforated sterile drape, chuck
- Shaver, shaver head, alcohol or betadine skin prep, marking pen, ruler, gauze
- 2–0 vicryl (10-pack), 3–0 monocryl (× 2), dermabond, 2–0 silk (× 1)
- Sterile flush (× 2), 23-gauge needle, tegaderm with chlorhexidine gluconate, regular tegaderm (× 3)
- Optional: paraffin bee's wax, cautery

In addition to standard ventriculostomy catheters, there are several ventriculostomy catheters on the market that are impregnated with antibiotics, usually rifampin. Studies have shown decreased risk of infection with these devices.[1] Drug allergies should be reviewed prior to use of an antibiotic-impregnated catheter.

1.6 Technique

1.6.1 Preparation

- Measure catheter trajectory, scalp thickness, skull thickness, and distance to the lateral ventricle on computed tomography (CT) of the head. A coronal plane reconstruction is preferred if available (see ▶ Fig. 1.6).
- Review results of relevant laboratory studies.

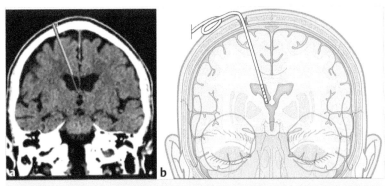

Fig. 1.6 Coronal measurement of ventricular drain depth. (Reproduced from Operative Procedure. In: Ullman J, Raksin PB. Atlas of Emergency Neurosurgery. 1st Edition. Thieme; 2015.)

1.6.2 Medications

- Oxygen should be administered via face mask if the patient is not intubated.
- Antibiotics with gram positive coverage are used for skin flora prophylaxis. Cefazolin is used most commonly. If using a cephalosporin, the medication should be administered as an intravenous (IV) push 5 minutes prior to incision. Administration of additional prophylactic antibiotics beyond this single peri-procedural dose is not recommended.[2]
- Antihypertensive agents should be used to maintain the systolic blood pressure less than 140 mm Hg during and immediately after the procedure. The calcium channel blocker nicardipine is most commonly used due to rapid action and ease of titration. Nitroprusside should not be used as it will cause an increase in ICP.
- Sedation is usually accomplished with propofol, midazolam, and fentanyl, all of which will confer additional antihypertensive effects.
- Lidocaine with or without epinephrine can be used for local anesthesia.

1.6.3 Positioning/Equipment Setup

- Position the patient supine with the head of the bed at 20 degrees. The patient's head should slightly overhang the top of bed. If there is a headboard on the bed it should be removed. The bed height should be adjusted for operator comfort.
- Place a chuck under the head of the bed.
- An open trash can should be positioned within reach.

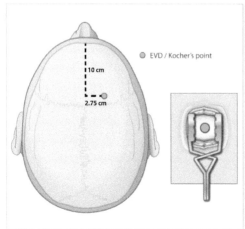

Fig. 1.7 Kocher's point. (Modified with permission from Operative Procedure. In: Ullman J, Raksin PB. Atlas of Emergency Neurosurgery. 1st Edition. Thieme; 2015.)

- A surgical headlight is usually not required, but all available room lights should be turned on.
- Shave the scalp widely.
- Wipe the shaved area of the scalp with alcohol.
- Dry the scalp and clearly mark the midline.
- Mark Kocher's point by measuring 10 cm posterior from glabella and 2.75 cm off midline (usually to the right side unless contraindicated) (see ▶ Fig. 1.7).
- Draw a line from Kocher's point to the ipsilateral medial canthus.
- Draw a line from Kocher's point to a point 1 cm anterior to ipsilateral tragus.
- These lines define the planes of insertion for the ventricular drain (see ▶ Fig. 1.8).
- Mark a 1-cm longitudinal stab incision centered on Kocher's point.
- Apply sterile prep to the scalp.
- Inject local anesthetic/epinephrine at the incision site, tunneling site, and lateral to incision for hemostasis (see ▶ Fig. 1.9).
- Open the cranial access kit on a table next to the bed to create a sterile field.
- Open all additional supplies onto the sterile field.
- Don a sterile gown, cap, facemask, and gloves.
- Place a large sterile drape under the patient's head while an assistant elevates the head from the base of the neck (see ▶ Fig. 1.10).
- Place a perforated sterile drape centered over Kocher's point.
- A second set of sterile gloves can be placed over the first at this point for additional sterility and operator protection.
- Flush the drainage collection system tubing with sterile saline.
- The ventricular catheter should also be irrigated.

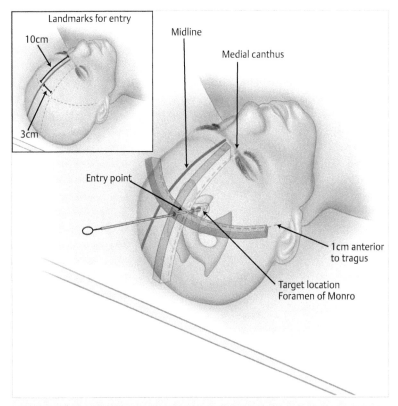

Fig. 1.8 Operator's view of head with planes depicting trajectory of catheter.

1.6.4 Procedure

- Make a 1 cm longitudinal incision with a #10 blade scalpel.
- Strip the periosteum at site of the burr hole using a mosquito clamp (see ▶ Fig. 1.11).
- Set the drill guard based on the combined thickness of the scalp and skull as measured from the coronal CT recon. Usually, this is approximately 1.5 cm.
- Drill a burr hole in plane with lines to the medial canthus and 1 cm anterior to the tragus. This should be roughly perpendicular to the scalp.
- There will be stiff resistance while drilling through the outer table of the skull, minimal resistance while drilling though the diploic bone, and maximum resistance while drilling through the inner table (see ▶ Fig. 1.12).
- Once the drill has engaged the inner table, slight counter pressure can be applied, pulling the drill back very slightly while the crank mechanism

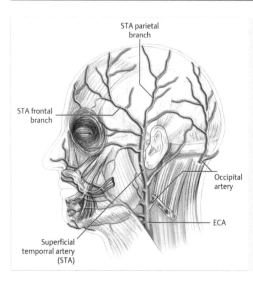

Fig. 1.9 Direction of blood supply to scalp. (Reproduced from Sekhar L, Fessler R, Hrsg. Atlas of Neurosurgical Techniques: Brain, Volume 2. 2nd Edition. Thieme; 2015.)

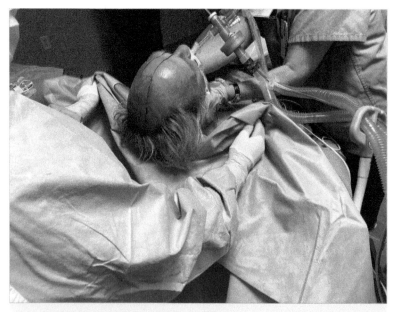

Fig. 1.10 Elevating head and placing drape.

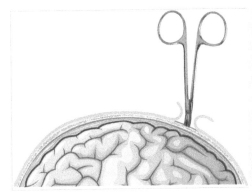

Fig. 1.11 Stripping of periosteum using mosquito clamp.

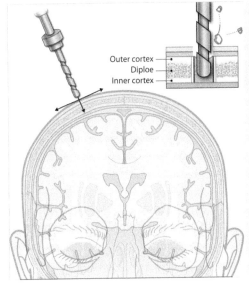

Outer cortex
Diploe
Inner cortex

Fig. 1.12 Burr hole trephination using a twist drill. (Reproduced from Operative Procedure. In: Ullman J, Raksin PB. Atlas of Emergency Neurosurgery. 1st Edition. Thieme; 2015.)

rotates the drill bit pulling it forward through the inner table. In conjunction with the drill guard, this will prevent "plunging" of the drill.

- Irrigate bone fragments out of the incision using a sterile saline flush.
- Confirm that the systolic blood pressure is less than 140 mm Hg. Administer additional propofol or nicardipine if needed.
- Insert the sharp end of the trochar into the wound and palpate the dura. Puncture the dura taking care not to insert the trochar more than 1 cm beyond the dural opening.
- Examine the ventricular catheter to confirm that the stylet is advanced to the catheter tip and that measurement markings on the catheter are visible.

- Pass catheter in the plane with the lines to the medial canthus and 1 cm anterior to the tragus. This should be approximately perpendicular to the scalp.
- An "ependymal pop" may be felt at a depth of around 4.5 cm, indicating entry into the ventricle.
- The target depth is ideally determined by measurement from the CT scan.
- In most adults, a depth of 6.5 to 7.0 cm at the skin will be appropriate.
- Once the catheter has been inserted to the target depth, the stylet is removed.
- There should be brisk flow of CSF from the catheter if it is situated appropriately.
- The ICP can be visually estimated by raising and lowering the distal end of the catheter to determine the height at which CSF continues to flow.
- CSF can be therapeutically drained at this stage if ICP reduction is emergently required.
- If necessary, a sample of CSF can be directly drained into collection vials for laboratory analysis.
- Connect the catheter to the blunt end of the trochar.
- Immobilize catheter at skull with a finger or rubber shod.
- Pass the trochar subcutaneously at least 5 cm. (It may be helpful to bend the trochar slightly prior to tunneling.)
- The direction of tunneling is usually posterior but will vary based on anticipated future procedures (see Expert Suggestions).
- Grasp the sharp end of the trochar with a hemostat and pull the trochar and redundant catheter out through the tunneling exit site, taking care not to pull the proximal end of the catheter back from the skull.
- Cut the catheter at the blunt end of the trochar and confirm appropriate flow of CSF.
- Place a cap on the catheter.
- Secure the cap with a 2–0 silk tie.
- Close the skin with one or two simple interrupted 3–0 monocryl stitches.
- Dermabond can be applied over the suture line.
- Secure catheter with a "Roman Sandal" 2–0 silk suture, and a strain-relief loop (see ▶ Fig. 1.13).
- Confirm CSF flow again.
- Attach the distal tubing to the collection system.
- Ensure that the collection tubing stopcock valves are occluded until the collection system is set to an appropriate height.
- Dress the catheter exit site with a chlorhexidine gluconate tegaderm. The catheter tubing can be secured to the patient's scalp, neck, and shoulder with additional tegaderms.

1.6.5 Alternative Approaches

Alternative approaches can be used if the standard frontal Kocher's approach is contraindicated. Several alternative approaches are described in Table 1.1 and depicted in ▶ Fig. 1.14.

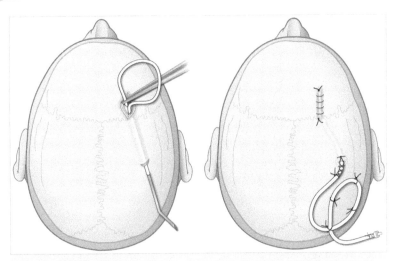

Fig. 1.13 Tunneling and anchoring of catheter. (Reproduced from Ullman J, Raksin PB. Atlas of Emergency Neurosurgery. 1st Edition. Thieme; 2015.)

Table 1.1 Alternative starting points and trajectories for ventricular drains

Eponym	Starting point	Trajectory
Frazier's Point	3 cm lateral to midline, 6 cm superior to inion	Toward contralateral medial canthus, ependyma should be reached at 4 cm, can be soft passed to 8 cm
Dandy's Point	2 cm lateral to midline, 3 cm superior to inion	Perpendicular to skull, slightly superior, ependyma should be reached at 4 cm, can be soft passed to 8 cm
Keen's Point	3 cm superior to pinna, 3 cm posterior to pinna	Perpendicular to skull, ependyma should be reached at 4 cm, can be soft passed to 8 cm

1.7 Complications

1.7.1 Infection

Infection is the most common clinically significant complicatifon of ventricular drain insertion. Most series report infection rates of around 8%.[3] Such infections can have serious consequences, resulting in hydrocephalus, neurologic decline, or death. The risk of infections can be minimized by employing meticulous sterile technique, administering a single dose of peri-procedural prophylactic antibiotics, using an antibiotic-coated catheter, tunneling the catheter

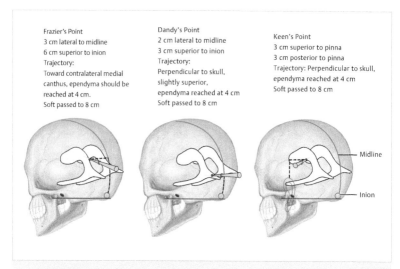

Frazier's Point
3 cm lateral to midline
6 cm superior to inion
Trajectory:
Toward contralateral medial
canthus, ependyma should be
reached at 4 cm.
Soft passed to 8 cm

Dandy's Point
2 cm lateral to midline
3 cm superior to inion
Trajectory:
Perpendicular to skull,
slightly superior,
ependyma reached at 4 cm
Soft passed to 8 cm

Keen's Point
3 cm superior to pinna
3 cm posterior to pinna
Trajectory: Perpendicular to skull,
ependyma reached at 4 cm
Soft passed to 8 cm

Midline

Inion

Fig. 1.14 Starting sites for Frazier's, Dandy's, and Keen's points.

subcutaneously at least 5 cm from the burr hole, minimizing manipulation of the CSF collection tubing system, and removing the ventricular drain as early as clinically feasible.

1.7.2 Hemorrhage

Reported hemorrhage rates following EVD insertion vary in the literature from 5 to 33%.[4] The rate of clinically detectable hemorrhage has been reported as 2.5%.[5] The risk of hemorrhage can be mitigated by correcting coagulopathy, thrombocytopenia, and hypertension prior to insertion. Surgical technique can also influence the hemorrhage rate. Care should be taken to avoid dural violation with the twist drill. The dural opening should be performed using the trochar without passing the trochar any deeper than necessary to pierce the dura. Consistent use of landmarks to guide catheter placement will assist with accuracy, thereby decreasing the number of catheter passes and tract hemorrhages.

1.7.3 Upward Herniation

Upward herniation refers to the expulsion of cerebellar tissue superiorly through the tentorial incisura resulting in compression of the midbrain. Although controversial and rarely observed, this phenomenon is believed to occur in the setting of posterior fossa swelling (due to mass lesion or stroke) when the opposing pressure of the supratentorial brain is rapidly reduced by decompression of the ventricular system. When there is concern for possible upward herniation, care should be taken to avoid excessive removal of CSF.

1.7.4 Aneurysm Re-rupture

When a ventricular drain is placed in the setting of aneurysmal subarachnoid hemorrhage, there is a theoretical risk of precipitating re-rupture of the aneurysm by lowering the pressure of the CSF space and thereby raising the transmural pressure gradient across the wall of the aneurysm. This complication is best avoided by ensuring appropriate blood pressure control prior to drain insertion.

1.7.5 Motor Cortex Injury

Damage to the motor cortex can occur when a ventricular drain is placed in an inappropriately posterior position. This complication can be avoided by ensuring the burr hole site is at least 3 cm anterior to the coronal suture.

1.7.6 Superior Sagittal Sinus Injury

Injury to the superior sagittal sinus results from medial placement of a ventricular drain. This potentially fatal complication can be avoided by carefully marking the midline, selecting a burr hole site at least 2.5 cm lateral to the midline, and holding the twist drill firmly to avoid migration of the drill tip while beginning the burr hole.

1.8 Expert Suggestions/Troubleshooting

1.8.1 Scalp Bleeding

Excessive scalp bleeding can pose a challenge since most ventricular drains are placed outside of the operating room (OR) without readily available electrocautery. The risk of transecting a scalp artery can be minimized by using a small stab incision. Injecting local anesthetic with epinephrine will result in vasoconstriction. This is especially helpful if injected several minutes prior to incision. When bleeding from a scalp artery cannot be stopped with manual compression, a stitch can be thrown adjacent to the incision (on the lateral side where the blood supply originates) to tie off the bleeding vessel. Alternatively, the incision can be lengthened to allow for insertion of a self-retaining retractor which will stop the bleeding by compressing and stretching the tissues.

Table 1.2 Preferred tunneling direction for given future procedures

Future procedure	Tunneling direction
Hemicraniectomy	Posterolateral
Bifrontal craniectomy	Posterior
Suboccipital craniectomy	Lateral
Ipsilateral craniotomy	Contralateral
Aneurysm clipping—unknown laterality	Posterior

1.8.2 Entry Site

Most commonly, ventricular drains are placed on the right side. When there is a strong possibility that the patient will need a right-sided craniotomy (i.e., right-sided mass lesion or aneurysm), the drain entry site should be on the left.

1.8.3 Tunneling Direction

Similar to selecting an appropriate entry site, the need for future procedures must be considered when tunneling the drain. Although this is a case by case determination, the general rules are described in ▶ Table 1.2.

1.8.4 Fracture Lines/Cranial Defects

A preoperative CT scan should be evaluated on bone windows to check for any fracture lines, burr holes, or other cranial defects prior to selecting an insertion site.

1.8.5 Ventricular Collapse

In patients with diffuse cerebral edema and elevated ICP, the ependymal walls may collapse around a ventricular catheter after draining only a few milliliters of CSF. When the ventricle collapses, drainage of CSF will stop, creating the misleading impression that the catheter has become displaced from the ventricle. In this situation, the catheter should not be repositioned and a CT scan should be obtained to confirm intraventricular placement. However, if CSF flow stops after insertion when preoperative imaging demonstrated larger ventricles, the system must be interrogated prior to breaking the sterile field. If the drain is secured with a stitch, this should be released to ensure that the catheter is not kinked. If this does not restore flow, the catheter should be removed and reinserted.

References

[1] Zabramski JM, Whiting D, Darouiche RO, et al. Efficacy of antimicrobial-impregnated external ventricular drain catheters: a prospective, randomized, controlled trial. J Neurosurg. 2003; 98(4): 725–730

[2] Fried HI, Nathan BR, Rowe AS, et al. The insertion and management of external ventricular drains: an evidence-based consensus statement: a statement for healthcare professionals from the Neurocritical Care Society. Neurocrit Care. 2016; 24(1):61–81

[3] Lozier AP, Sciacca RR, Romagnoli MF, Connolly ES, Jr. Ventriculostomy-related infections: a critical review of the literature. Neurosurgery. 2002; 51(1):170–181, discussion 181–182

[4] Kakarla UK, Kim LJ, Chang SW, Theodore N, Spetzler RF. Safety and accuracy of bedside external ventricular drain placement. Neurosurgery. 2008; 63(1) Suppl 1:ONS162–ONS166, discussion ONS166–ONS167

[5] Maniker AH, Vaynman AY, Karimi RJ, Sabit AO, Holland B. Hemorrhagic complications of external ventricular drainage. Neurosurgery. 2006; 59(4) Suppl 2:ONS419–ONS424, discussion ONS424–ONS425

2 Shunt Tap and Shunt Externalization

Yehuda Herschman

Abstract

A shunt tap or externalization can be performed in various clinical scenarios – most commonly shunt obstruction or infection. Here the following topics related to shunt tap and externalization are discussed in detail: relevant anatomy and physiology, indications/contraindications, equipment, technique, complications, and expert suggestions.

Keywords: shunt, shunt tap, externalization, CSF, shunt infection

2.1 Introduction

A shunt is a tubular system, for cerebrospinal fluid (CSF) diversion, that is composed of a proximal catheter, valve, distal catheter, and sometimes a reservoir. It allows for the alleviation of elevated intracranial pressure (ICP), particularly hydrocephalus, by diverting CSF from the ventricular system to a distal terminus. The most common terminus for a shunt is the peritoneal cavity: however, the pleura or right ventricle of the heart are often used as a secondary option as well. ▶ Fig. 2.1 depicts a ventriculoperitoneal shunt system. The etiologies of hydrocephalus are many and varied and are beyond the scope of this chapter.

Once a neurosurgeon implants a shunt, many complications may arise in both an acute setting or many years after the initial surgery. The most common complication of a shunt is malfunction. The reason for the malfunction is of vital importance to the clinician in order to ascertain how to properly treat and correct the underlying etiology for the "shunt failure." A detailed history and physical examination, including an examination for papilledema is key. Of note, patients who present with shunt failure, either in the ambulatory or emergency setting, will most often re-present with their initial symptoms prior to having the shunting procedure, many of which are associated with elevated ICP including papilledema, headache, vomiting, diplopia, impaired up-gaze, coma, seizure, or imbalance.

In the process of working up a shunt malfunction, one must determine whether it is due to infection, hardware failure (e.g., fractured hardware), proximal catheter obstruction, obstruction of the shunt valve, or distal catheter obstruction. Critical to this workup is the following imaging: computed tomography (CT) of the head or magnetic resonance imaging (MRI) of the brain, anteroposterior (AP) and lateral skull X-rays, chest X-ray, and abdominal X-ray

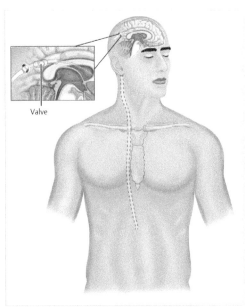

Fig. 2.1 Schematic of ventriculoperitoneal shunt system.

Valve

(if the distal terminus is in the peritoneum). Having prior imaging from previous encounters, in particular one that allows visualization of the ventricular system is extremely useful. The skull film enables the clinician to determine what type of valve the shunt system has (▶ Fig. 2.2), whether it has a reservoir, and where they are in relation to skull anatomy. Additionally, the X-rays should be reviewed for any fractures of the hardware, disconnections, or kinking of the tubing that could lead to malfunction (▶ Fig. 2.3). One may also undertake a nuclear shunt study, or "shunt-o-gram," which entails injection of a radio-isotope into the shunt system to determine if there is proper flow. If prior imaging and a nuclear shunt study are unavailable, then the provider must rely on clinical judgment. A shunt tap or externalization can be performed for diagnostic and therapeutic purposes in the setting of shunt malfunction.

2.2 Relevant Anatomy and Physiology

A shunt system allows for diversion of CSF from the ventricles of the brain to other areas of the body. When the pressure in the ventricular system, or ICP, is greater than that of the opening pressure setting of the valve, fluid will flow from the proximal ventricular catheter through the system to the terminus of the distal catheter. The body then absorbs this excess of CSF in the cavity into which it is deposited. A more detailed description of CSF physiology can be

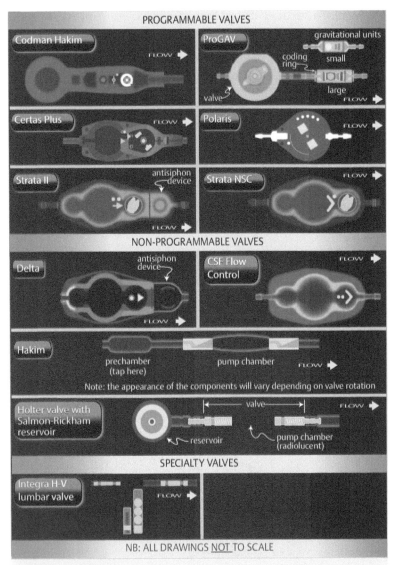

Fig. 2.2 Schematic of common valve systems. Reproduced with permission from Greenberg M, ed. Handbook of Neurosurgery. 8th Edition. Thieme; 2016.

found in the ventriculostomy chapter (see Chapter 1 External Ventricular Drain).

Most often, the system begins with a proximal ventricular catheter either frontally, near Kocher's point, or posteriorly near Keen's or Frazier's point (see Chapter 1 External Ventricular Drain). This proximal catheter is then attached to a valve, with or without a reservoir, and a distal catheter is connected to the valve or reservoir. The shunt valve most often sits on the flat surface of the skull. This is important for shunt programming and shunt tapping in order to identify the valve by palpation. The course of the distal catheter most commonly runs in the anterior lateral portion of the neck, riding over the sterno-cleidomastoid and then continuing over the clavicle prior to depositing either in the pleura or peritoneum. For those patients who have a ventricular atrial shunt, the distal catheter is placed in either the facial vein or the internal jugular vein within the neck. It is of vital importance to know the course of the distal catheter, especially if one is to externalize the shunt.

2.3 Indications—Shunt Tap (▶ Fig. 2.3)

Patients who have shunts may have several reasons to have their shunt systems evaluated. Often times, if one is concerned as to whether the shunt is working properly or not a shunt tap may be most useful.

The placement of a small gauge needle, 23-gauge butterfly needle most preferably, allows for accessing the shunt system. By doing so the clinician must realize that there is a risk of introducing potential infection to a sterile environment. This risk must be weighed carefully when considering the need for a shunt tap in evaluating a shunt system.

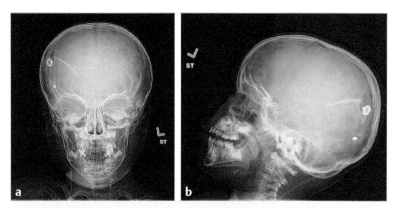

Fig. 2.3 (a, b) X ray of catheter disconnection. (Reproduced with permission from Ullman J and Raksin PB. Atlas of Emergency Neurosurgery. © Thieme 2015.)

There are two primary reasons to tap a shunt: first, to obtain access to the CSF, and second, to determine if there is proper flow of CSF. These two categories can be further subdivided. By obtaining access to CSF via shunt tapping, one can easily take a CSF sample to be evaluated for microbiological purposes for infectious workup. With this access to the shunt system one can also use this opportunity to administer intrathecal medications (i.e., antibiotics or medications).

During workup for possible shunt failure, information from a shunt tap can be most useful in helping to determine if there is proper flow or if there is an obstruction within the system. This can be done either by injecting a radioisotope into the system or by manually evaluating the flow (this will be discussed later in this chapter).

2.4 Contraindications—Shunt Tap

The following are relative contraindications to performing a shunt tap:
• Scalp infection
• Nonaccessible shunt valve or lack of shunt reservoir
• Bacteremia

2.5 Equipment—Shunt Tap

The following equipment is needed for a shunt tap:
• 23-gauge butterfly needle
• 5 mL syringe
• Sterile saline
• Manometer
• Hair clipper
• Sterile skin prep
• Cap, mask, gown, sterile gloves, and sterile drapes

2.6 Technique—Shunt Tap

2.6.1 Preparation

Review relevant imaging, particularly the shunt series, to determine where the shunt valve lies.

2.6.2 Medications

Medications are not routinely administered when performing a shunt tap.

2.6.3 Positioning/Equipment Setup

- The patient should be in the supine position on a bed or a stretcher with the head turned toward the contralateral side of the shunt valve.
- The valve is then palpated underneath the skin.
- A minimal amount of hair is shaven over the area of the shunt valve.
- The skin overlying the shunt valve is then cleaned with alcohol and chlorhexidine gluconate.
- Dress in a sterile gown, gloves, cap, and mask.
- Sterile drapes should then be placed around the area of the shaven hair.
- Open the sterile 23-gauge butterfly needle, sterile saline flush, and 5 mL syringe on a sterile field.

2.6.4 Procedure

- A 23-gauge butterfly needle is placed into the valve or reservoir of the shunt without the syringe attached, as depicted in ▶ Fig. 2.4.
- The end of the tubing from the butterfly needle is then held carefully and elevated above the patient's head to determine if there is active flow. The ICP can be visually estimated based upon the height of the fluid column in the tubing.
- A mobile meniscus indicates that the proximal catheter is functioning. It would be difficult from this shunt tap alone to determine whether the distal catheter is functioning properly.
- If there is a significant flow while the tubing is held above the patient's head, this would seem to indicate possible elevated ICP and a distal obstruction.
- If no flow is seen then an empty 5 mL syringe can be connected to gently aspirate from the valve. If nothing can be aspirated then the shunt system must be fully interrogated in the operating room.

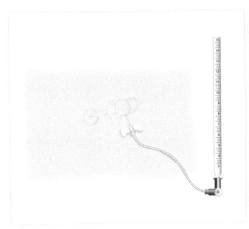

Fig. 2.4 Manometer assessment of intracranial pressure (ICP).

- This technique can also be used when attempting to obtain a CSF culture for a shunt infection workup.
- When needed, either medication or radioisotope can be injected into the shunt system at the time of the shunt tap.
- For a more accurate reading, a manometer with a three-way stopcock can be connected to the 23-gauge butterfly needle to determine more clearly a mobile meniscus and the opening pressure which equals the ICP, as depicted in ▶ Fig. 2.4.
- One can also attempt to test for distal obstruction through the use of a shunt tap. With the 23-gauge butterfly needle in place, the provider must also depress the proximal portion of the shunt valve. By doing so this obstructs the proximal flow and isolates the distal portion of the system. Once this is done, gentle infusion of sterile saline can be "pushed through" to the distal system. If the saline flows easily and freely, then the likelihood of a distal obstruction is minimal. However, if significant resistance is encountered, then this is a strong indication of a distal obstruction within the shunt system.

2.7 Indications—Shunt Externalization

Many of the indications to externalize a shunt are very much dependent upon the workup of shunt failure. If the patient presents with clinical and radiological shunt failure, and it is clear from the imaging studies that there is a distal fracture of hardware (distal to the valve) then urgent externalization of the shunt, or distal revision of the shunt, is warranted. Externalization of the shunt allows for the continuation of proper CSF flow and ICP control. In the event that a workup reveals a proximal shunt malfunction (proximal to the shunt valve and inclusive of the valve) then a shunt externalization would be contraindicated.

The two primary indications for shunt externalization are: distal shunt failure and shunt infection. Distal shunt failure may be the result of different etiologies that include fracture of distal hardware, abdominal or pelvic pseudocyst in peritoneal shunts, symptomatic pleural effusion in pleural shunts, and abdominal/pelvic complications not related to the shunt or its implantation. When dealing with a shunt that is infected it may be of benefit to externalize the shunt while cultures and susceptibilities of the CSF become final in order to determine the proper course. At that point, depending on the specific organism, one may continue externalization while on the appropriate antibiotic regimen until the CSF is deemed to be clear of infection. Once the CSF is cleared the entire shunt system should be revised. Alternatively, the entire shunt system can be removed from the outset and replaced with an external ventricular drain during the period of antibiotic therapy until the patient is cleared to have a new shunt system placed.

Additionally, if there is a concern for infection at the terminus that is unrelated to the shunt itself (i.e., open abdomen, abdominal sepsis, or other abdominal catastrophe), a shunt externalization may be considered in order to prevent an ascending ventriculitis.

2.8 Contraindications—Shunt Externalization

The following are contraindications to shunt externalization:
• Proximal shunt malfunction
• Acute neurologic decline
• Uncertainty as to where the shunt is malfunctioning

2.9 Equipment—Shunt Externalization

• Ventricular catheter package (contains catheter connector to attach to collection system)
• CSF collection system burette
• Lidocaine with epinephrine
• Cap, mask, gown, sterile gloves (×2), perforated sterile drape, and chuck
• 2–0 vicryl (10-pack), 3–0 monocryl (×2), dermabond, 2–0 silk (×1), 2–0 nylon
• Sterile flush (×2), 23-gauge needle, tegaderm with chlorhexidine gluconate, and regular tegaderm (×2)
• Hair clipper
• Single-use instrument set including scissors, mosquito clamp, forceps, and needle driver
• #15 blade

2.10 Technique—Shunt Externalization

2.10.1 Preparation

• Review of the imaging, particularly the shunt series, to determine where the shunt catheter sits in relation to the clavicle or other landmarks.
• Review relevant laboratory studies.

2.10.2 Medications

• Oxygen should be administered via face mask if the patient is not intubated.
• Antibiotics with gram positive coverage are used for skin flora prophylaxis. Cefazolin is used most commonly. If using a cephalosporin, the medication should be administered as an IV push 5 minutes prior to incision.
• Sedation is usually accomplished with propofol, midazolam, and fentanyl.
• Lidocaine with or without epinephrine can be used for local anesthesia.

2.10.3 Positioning/Equipment Setup

- In this section we will describe a shunt externalization at the clavicle. However, one can externalize a distal shunt catheter at any point along its tract that is distal to the shunt valve.
- The patient should be positioned supine on a bed with the head in a neutral position.
- The area of the shunt catheter riding over the clavicle should be palpated if possible. It may not be possible to palpate in those patients with significant amount of tissue.
- If the patient has hair overlying the clavicle it is shaved widely.
- The area is then thoroughly cleaned with alcohol and chlorhexidine gluconate.
- A horizontal line is then marked out across the clavicle in the expected area of the shunt catheter.
- Dress in a sterile gown, gloves, cap, and mask.
- Sterile drapes should then be placed around the area of the shaven hair.

2.10.4 Procedure

- Local anesthesia is infiltrated to the skin overlying the clavicle in the marked area.
- The equipment for the shunt externalization is then placed on a sterile field.
- Using the #15 blade, a 2-cm horizontal incision is made over the shunt tubing at the level of the clavicle. Care should be taken not to cut through all layers of the dermis.
- Blunt dissection using a mosquito clamp should then be carefully performed so as not to damage the distal shunt catheter.
- Once the catheter is visually identified place the clamp beneath it and pull up on the distal aspect of the catheter, as depicted in ▶ Fig. 2.5.
- If the distal catheter comes easily, pull it up and out through the incision.
- If there is resistance when pulling on the distal catheter, do not remove it.
- At this point place the clamp on the catheter below the point of the clavicle.
- Cut the catheter with a scissor below the clamp.
- Attach the portion of catheter that is held within the clamp to the connecter (found in the ventricular catheter package) and place a tie to secure it to the catheter.
- At this point it should be seen if there is free flow of CSF. If there is not, the patient must be brought to the operating room for a shunt revision. If there is free flow of CSF, then one may proceed with the remainder of the externalization procedure.
- Place a cap (in the ventricular catheter package) on the proximal catheter so that CSF does not continue to drain.
- Close the incision around the catheter.
- Using 2–0 vicryl sutures, close the dermis with inverted interrupted sutures, taking care not to damage or entangle the catheter.

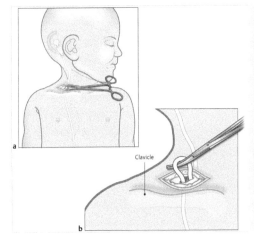

Fig. 2.5 Shunt externalization at clavicle. (Reproduced from Operative Procedure. In: Ullman J, Raksin PB. Atlas of Emergency Neurosurgery. 1st Edition. Thieme; 2015.)

- Close the skin with a running 3–0 monocryl.
- The catheter that is now external to the skin is secured to the skin with a 2–0 nylon suture in roman sandal fashion.
- At this point the CSF collection system burette should be flushed with sterile saline and then connected to the now externalized catheter.
- The incision is dressed with sterile gauze and tegaderm.
- The burette is attached to a pole next to the patient's bed. The height of the burette can be set anywhere at or below the level of the tragus as the shunt valve will regulate the flow of CSF.

2.11 Complications

2.11.1 Infection

One of the greatest concerns when tapping or externalizing a shunt is the risk of introducing infection to a sterile shunt system. Though the likelihood of introducing an infection via shunt tap is extremely low aseptic conditions should certainly be followed.

2.11.2 Catheter Retraction

When performing a shunt externalization, there is a possibility that the proximal portion may retract upward and the catheter can be lost into deeper tissue that cannot be explored at the bedside. For that reason, one should try to create a small loop and place a clamp on the catheter prior to cutting it (▶ Fig. 2.5). In the event that the catheter retracts, it is not advisable to explore further at the bedside. Rather the entire system should be interrogated and explored in the operating room.

2.11.3 Air Lock of Shunt System

One must be careful to avoid introducing air into the shunt system while performing a shunt tap or externalization, although this is more likely to happen with a shunt tap. If air enters the system, it may then obstruct the flow of CSF leading to shunt failure. Making certain not to inject any air into the shunt valve and system is of the utmost importance.

2.12 Expert Suggestions/Troubleshooting

2.12.1 Inability to Tap Shunt Valve

In some instances, a shunt cannot be tapped. If you find that you have tried to insert the needle over the palpated valve but could not enter the valve, then perhaps this is a valve that cannot be tapped. It is of great importance to review the imaging to determine, if possible, what type of shunt valve is implanted and whether one can access it via a needle.

2.12.2 Distal Catheter Resistance

It is possible that during an externalization of a shunt when attempting to remove the distal portion of the catheter, resistance may be encountered. This is not entirely uncommon and may also be the potential reason for shunt failure. It is advised not to continue to attempt to remove it and rather abandon the distal catheter in situ and proceed with the remainder of the externalization.

2.12.3 Partial Retraction of the Shunt Catheter

When externalizing a shunt, it is possible that the more proximal portion, which is to be externalized, may retract up toward the neck. For this reason, it is advisable to place a clamp on the catheter prior to dividing it. However, even with a clamp it may still retract. The clamp at this point may allow you to maintain a hold on the now partially retracted catheter. This can be salvaged. In order to do so one needs a straight connector and a ventricular catheter. At this point one can cut off the distal end of the ventriculostomy catheter (pointed end) to create a hollow catheter open at both ends. Next, place the straight connector on one of the ends of the ventriculostomy catheter and secure it with a tie. One may now attach the other end of the straight connector to the partially retracted shunt catheter at the clavicle. Be sure to secure this end with a tie as well, otherwise it will retract and detach from the ventricular catheter. From this point one proceeds with attaching the locking cap and connecting to the burette as described earlier in this chapter.

3 Lumbar Puncture

R. Nick Hernandez, Neil Majmundar, and Amna Sheikh

Abstract

This chapter will discuss the indications and contraindications, relevant anatomy, technique, complications, and tips for performing a lumbar puncture.

Keywords: lumbar puncture, technique, neurointensive care

3.1 Introduction

Lumbar puncture (LP) is a procedure performed to access the cerebrospinal fluid (CSF), either for diagnostic or therapeutic purposes. A long, thin needle is used to puncture the skin in the lower back and the needle is advanced until it punctures the spinal dura. The procedure therefore provides access to the lumbar CSF space. This allows direct measurement of the pressure within the CSF space and collection of CSF for gross and laboratory analysis. This chapter will discuss the relevant anatomy, indications and contraindications, equipment required, technique for safe LP performance, and related complications.

3.2 Relevant Anatomy

3.2.1 Cerebrospinal Fluid

The majority of CSF is produced by the choroid plexus located intracranially within the ventricular system. CSF flows through the ventricles and exits the ventricular system via the foramina of Luschka and Magendie, where it enters the subarachnoid space to surround the brain and spinal cord. CSF is reabsorbed via the arachnoid granulations adjacent to the superior sagittal sinus[1] (▶ Fig. 3.1). The total volume of CSF at any given point in time is about 150 cc and the rate of CSF production is about 20 to 25 cc/hour, or 450 to 500 cc/day. This results in the resorption and regeneration of the total CSF volume three to four times daily. The ventricles contain only 20% of the total CSF volume at any given time with the remaining amount distributed within the cranial and spinal subarachnoid spaces and cisterns.[2] A large amount of CSF resides in the lumbar region; thus, CSF can be effectively accessed in the lumbar spine.

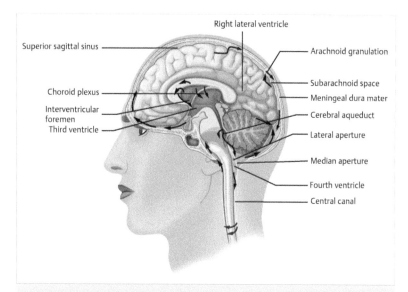

Fig. 3.1 Flow of cerebrospinal fluid (CSF) within the intraventricular system. CSF is generated by the choroid plexus and is reabsorbed into the superior sagittal sinus via the arachnoid granulations.

3.2.2 Lumbar Spine

In the adult patient, the spinal cord terminates as the conus medullaris at around the L1 level.[3] Below the conus medullaris, spinal nerve roots travel within the thecal sac surrounded by CSF to exit the spinal column via their respective neural foramina. Due to the termination of the spinal cord at the upper lumbar levels, there is no risk of injuring the spinal cord when the thecal sac is accessed at the lower lumbar levels in the vast majority of patients. ▶ Fig. 3.2 depicts the relevant anatomy of the lumbar spine.

3.3 Indications

There are several indications for obtaining access to the CSF space. These indications can be broken into four broad indications: (1) to obtain a CSF sample for laboratory analysis, (2) to measure the pressure within the neuraxis, (3) to perform therapeutic drainage of CSF, and (4) to administer medication.

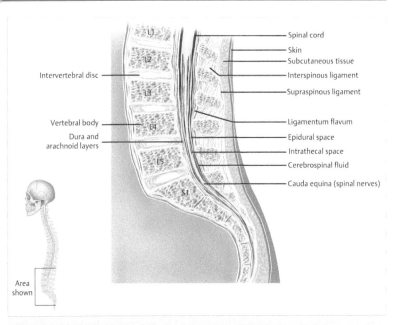

Fig. 3.2 Lumbar spinal anatomy.

3.3.1 Obtain a CSF Sample

The broadest indication for LP is to obtain a CSF specimen for analysis. A number of neurologic pathologies can be diagnosed with CSF sampling, including viral or bacterial infections, primary central nervous system (CNS) or metastatic malignancies, some neurodegenerative conditions, and autoimmune diseases. Gross examination of CSF includes clarity (clear vs. cloudy) and color (clear, yellow, red, etc.). In patients with a suspected diagnosis of subarachnoid hemorrhage (SAH) but a negative computed tomography (CT) of the head, CSF obtained via LP can be examined for the presence of xanthochromia, which would support the diagnosis of SAH.

3.3.2 Measure Pressure

Many neurologic diseases can result in elevated intracranial pressure (ICP), including meningitis, malignancies, ventriculoperitoneal shunt failure, idiopathic intracranial hypertension, communicating hydrocephalus, and trauma. Obtaining a pressure measurement of the CSF space often guides clinicians on the most appropriate course of treatment, such as the use of hypertonic saline or the need for shunt revision surgery. LP with the patient in the lateral decubitus position can provide a real-time measurement of the pressure within the neuraxis and help guide clinicians on the best course of action.

3.3.3 Therapeutic Drainage

There are a number of indications for therapeutic drainage of CSF. In general, any instance of ICP crisis due to communicating hydrocephalus may be temporarily treated with LP and therapeutic drainage of CSF, such as a patient presenting with shunt failure who requires temporization prior to a definitive operative intervention (i.e., shunt revision surgery) as long as there is no obstruction to flow. Additionally, therapeutic drainage of CSF in patients with normal pressure hydrocephalus (NPH) or idiopathic intracranial hypertension (IIH) can aid in determining if such patients would benefit from permanent CSF shunting. In such patients, high-volume LP results in marked symptom improvement. Patients with cryptococcal meningitis often develop chronic communicating hydrocephalus. In such cases it may be necessary to perform daily LPs as a temporizing bridge to permanent ventriculoperitoneal shunting while antifungals are administered to clear the infection.

LP can be performed to access the CSF space for the purpose of administering medications. The most common scenario in which this would be done would be for the administration of iodinated contrast for the purpose of CT myelography imaging of the spine.

3.4 Contraindications

The following are relative contraindications to LP.

3.4.1 Intracranial Space-Occupying Lesion or Existing Brain Shift

In a patient with an intracranial space-occupying lesion(s) in which brain compression and elevated ICP are suspected or confirmed, there is concern that removal of CSF from the lumbar cistern may result in downward intracranial herniation. As described by van Crevel et al, "*the withdrawal of the CSF removes the stopper from below, thus adding to the effects of the compression from above, and increasing the brain shifts already present.*"[4] This downward herniation may result in compression of the brainstem as well as other critical neurovascular structures, and can result in significant morbidity or mortality. Clinical findings that should prompt CT scan of the head prior to LP include altered mental status, focal neurologic deficits, or comatose state. If the results of the CT are inconclusive or cannot definitively rule out a space-occupying lesion, advanced imaging with magnetic resonance imaging (MRI) should be pursued. Nevertheless, if the benefit outweighs the risk, a low-volume LP may be performed in such patients, taking care to remove the minimum amount of CSF needed and monitoring the patient closely following the procedure. Perhaps most illustrative is the case of acute bacterial meningitis (ABM), in which patients can present with severely altered mental status and ICP is often elevated, but rapid diagnosis is necessary to prevent the morbidity and mortality associated with untreated or delayed treatment of ABM.

Note that elevated ICP and/or papilledema alone, as in idiopathic intracranial hypertension, are not contraindications if present without an intracranial space-occupying mass.

3.4.2 Obstructive Hydrocephalus

Similar to the concern with intracranial space-occupying lesions, obstructive hydrocephalus results in isolated elevated ICP. Removal of CSF from the lumbar cistern can thus lead to downward herniation.

3.4.3 Coagulopathy/Clotting Dysfunction/Bleeding Disorder

There are a number of external and internal causes for bleeding dysfunction in patients that may require LP. These include pre-existing coagulopathies (e.g., hemophilia, von Willebrand disease, and liver failure), medication-induced dysfunction of the clotting cascade (e.g., warfarin, heparin, rivaroxaban, and argatroban) or of platelet function (aspirin, clopidogrel, etc.), recent thrombolytic therapy (e.g., tPA administered for acute ischemic stroke), and thrombocytopenia.

Nevertheless, if LP is determined to be necessary for the appropriate medical treatment of an individual patient, appropriate reversal agents or blood product(s) can be administered prior to the procedure. The incidence of LP-related spinal hematomas reported in the literature is extremely rare,[5,6] although the true incidence, anecdotally, is likely higher as not all cases are reported. Each case should be evaluated individually to determine the risk and benefit of performing LP in the presence of coagulopathy. If the benefit outweighs the risk of possible hematoma, and the patient and/or family has been counseled and understands the risks and would like to proceed with the procedure, LP can be performed.

3.4.4 Insertion Site Infection

In the presence of infection at the needle insertion site, LP should be avoided in order to prevent potential seeding of the CNS. Such infections would include superficial skin infection overlying the lumbar spine and/or deeper soft tissue infections or abscesses that would be in or near the trajectory of the LP needle. In these cases, access to the CSF should be sought elsewhere in the neuraxis.

3.5 Equipment

The majority of the equipment needed to perform an LP is contained within a pre-packaged LP kit (▶ Fig. 3.3). Additionally, sterile attire should be worn during the procedure. Below is a list of the necessary equipments:

- Sterile gown and gloves
- Mask and head bouffant
- Skin preparation (chloroprep, chlorhexidine, betadine, etc.)
- Sterile drapes
- Sterile gauze
- 1% lidocaine
- 10 cc syringe
- 23-gauge needle
- Spinal needle (preferably atraumatic)
- Three-way stopcock
- Manometer
- CSF collection tubes (four)
- Band-aid or occlusive adhesive dressing

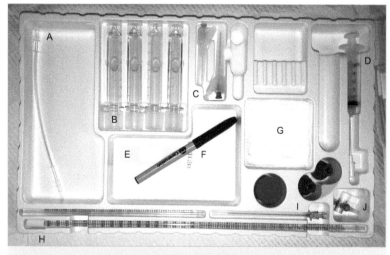

Fig. 3.3 Lumbar puncture (LP) kit. **(A)** Lengthening adapter. **(B)** Collection tubes. **(C)** Anesthetic needles. **(D)** Syringe. **(E)** Band-aid. **(F)** Marking pen. **(G)** Gauze. **(H)** Manometer. Note in this kit that the manometer comes as two separate pieces and must be assembled. **(I)** Spinal needle. **(J)** Three-way stopcock.

3.6 Technique

Prior to embarking on LP, relevant laboratory values should be reviewed, and if any coagulopathy exists, it should be corrected appropriately. Patients with altered mental status and/or focal neurologic deficits or with concern for intracranial space-occupying lesions should undergo CT scan of the head prior to LP. Diagnosis can often be made based on neuroimaging alone, precluding the need for LP. If the patient still requires an LP after the appropriate neuroimaging is completed, one must weigh the risks and benefits of performing the LP based upon clinical presentation, imaging findings, laboratory values, and the need for diagnosis.

3.6.1 Patient Positioning

The patient should be positioned in the lateral decubitus position. The hips and knees should be flexed as much as possible and the chin should touch the chest, much like the fetal position (▶ Fig. 3.4b). If the patient is compliant, the patient may be able to get into this position without assistance. In other cases, an assistant should stand opposite the operator to assist the patient with the positioning. This position results in widening of the lumbar interlaminar space, facilitating passage of the needle.

Alternatively, the patient may be positioned in the sitting position. The patient is positioned on the edge of the bed with his or her legs hanging off the bed. The patient is instructed to lean forward onto a table so as to flex the back

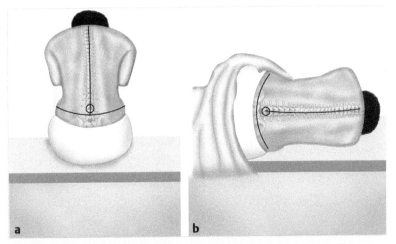

Fig. 3.4 (a) The sitting and (b) lateral decubitus positions. A line connecting the iliac crests approximates the L4 level and represents a good starting point for needle insertion.

and open the interlaminar space (▶ Fig. 3.4a). This position is often attempted if LP in the lateral decubitus position is unsuccessful. By positioning the patient in the sitting position, the lumbar thecal sac becomes a dependent position. CSF thus collects in the lumbar cistern and may improve the success rate of LP. One must note that pressure should not be measured in the seated position and if pressure is to be measured the patient should carefully be moved into the lateral decubitus position once the CSF space has been successfully accessed.

3.6.2 Preparation

The skin overlying the lumbar spine should be prepped and draped in sterile fashion. The operator should wear a cap and mask and don sterile gloves and a gown. Sterile drapes should be applied leaving the lumbar spine exposed. The iliac crest correlates roughly to the L4/L5 intervertebral space. By palpating the iliac crest and drawing a visual line from the iliac crest to the midline, the operator can identify a reasonable needle insertion site. The operator should then palpate over this area in the midline to identify the spinous processes and mark, with a marker or mentally, a point in the midline between the two spinous processes. At this point, 1% lidocaine anesthetic should be administered. Start by creating a small wheal in the skin. Advance the needle until bone is encountered and then inject more lidocaine. Numbing these areas first can help reduce or eliminate pain of the procedure, especially when the spinal needle encounters the bony anatomy which can be particularly painful.

While the anesthetic takes effect, the operator can set up the equipment from the LP kit. The operator should know where all the required equipment is prior to beginning the procedure to ensure efficient and sterile performance of the LP. One should not be fumbling to find the CSF collection tubes while there is CSF egress from the spinal needle. Identify and relocate the following items for easy access during the procedure: spinal needle, adapter, three-way stopcock, manometer, collection tubes, and gauze.

3.6.3 Needle Insertion

If available, an atraumatic spinal needle should be used which has been shown to decrease the risk of procedure-related complications compared to the conventional spinal needle[7] (▶ Fig. 3.5). Identify the bevel of the spinal needle. During insertion, the bevel should be facing up (toward the ceiling in the lateral decubitus position), parallel to the thecal sac. This orientation serves two purposes: to lower the risk of post-LP headache by entering the thecal sac in plane with the longitudinal fibers of the dura[8] and if a nerve root is encountered the root is more likely to be pushed away rather than cut. Insert the needle through the skin at the site where the local anesthetic was administered. If the patient feels significant pain, either allow more time for the anesthetic to

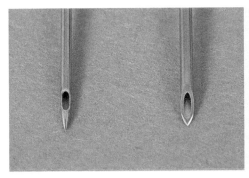

Fig. 3.5 Two commonly used spinal needles. *Left*: Atraumatic Sprotte needle (21-gauge) with a conical tip. *Right*: Quincke needle (20-gauge) with a sharp tip. (Reproduced from Wildemann, Brigitte et al. Laboratory Diagnosis in Neurology. Thieme Verlagsgruppe, Stuttgart, New York, Delhi, Rio; 2010.)

take effect or administer more. Systemic analgesia may also be administered. The starting trajectory should be parallel to the floor and approximately 30 degrees cranial, or parallel to the angle of the spinous processes. Advance the needle slowly taking care to feel the anatomy as the needle advances. The spinous process may be encountered, in which case the operator may "walk" the needle down the spinous process to the lamina if using a larger gauge spinal needle. If using a small gauge needle, it is best to withdraw and correct the angle of approach. Once the needle encounters the lamina, one can continue to "walk" or re-angle the needle until the interlaminar space is identified. One may not encounter any bone if the patient is optimally positioned. As the operator advances the needle, he or she may feel loss of resistance at several points. The first is often the supraspinous and interspinous ligaments followed by ligamentum flavum and lastly the dura (▶ Fig. 3.6). There is no harm in removing the inner stylet periodically to assess for CSF flow, but the needle should never be advanced without the stylet in place to avoid the delayed complication of spinal epidermoid cyst. Once the operator believes that the needle is in the lumbar cistern, the inner stylet is removed and CSF egress is confirmed. At this point, one should reintroduce the stylet to avoid CSF loss, and turn the needle so that the bevel is facing cranially.

3.6.4 Pressure Measurement

Assemble the manometer with the three-way stopcock attached at the base. Attach the stopcock to the spinal needle with the flow of CSF directed into the manometer (▶ Fig. 3.7). A flexible adapter can also be used to connect the needle to the stopcock. Allow the manometer to fill and record the opening pressure, noting that the meniscus will bounce with heartbeat and fluctuate with respiration. It is also good practice to record the closing pressure after the CSF specimen has been collected. Note that pressure recording must be performed when the patient is in the lateral decubitus position, as a pressure recorded in the sitting position will be artificially elevated due to the dependent position.

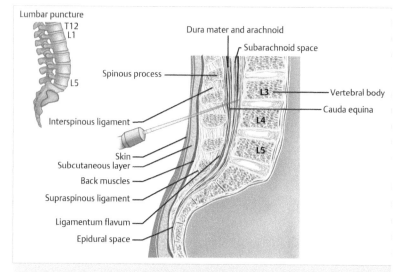

Fig. 3.6 The trajectory of the lumbar puncture (LP) needle through the lumbar spinal anatomy and final position of the needle in the lumbar cistern.

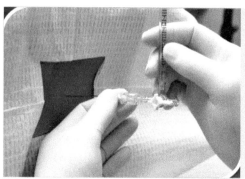

Fig. 3.7 Intracranial pressure measurement. The three-way stopcock has been assembled and attached to the end of the spinal needle. Courtesy: Gaumard Scientific.

3.6.5 CSF Collection

Assemble the collection tubes. If sending CSF to evaluate for SAH, be sure the tubes are labeled in order of CSF collection so that the red blood cell count can be distinguished the between tubes which will allow one to differentiate SAH from traumatic LP. Collect the appropriate amount of CSF required. Attaching the lengthening adapter to the spinal needle can aid in collection as the tubing is flexible and can be manipulated to facilitate drainage directly into the collection tubes,

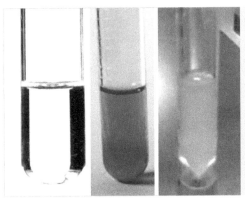

Fig. 3.8 Various cerebrospinal fluid (CSF) samples. It is important to document the color and clarity of the CSF sample.

whereas obtaining the dripping CSF from the spinal needle can be sometimes difficult depending on the angle of the needle. If a high-volume LP is being performed, one may remove 30 to 40 cc of CSF. Allow the CSF to spontaneously drip from the spinal needle; do not apply suction to the needle to obtain CSF faster. If during collection the CSF flow ceases or becomes slow, one may ask an assistant to place the patient's bed into reverse Trendelenburg, or carefully move the patient into the sitting position. This will facilitate CSF egress. One should note the color and clarity of the CSF (e.g., clear, yellow, red, and cloudy; ▶ Fig. 3.8). After collecting the CSF, make sure the tubes are sealed and appropriately labeled prior to sending to the laboratory.

3.6.6 Closure

Prior to removal of the spinal needle, the stylet should be reinserted to decrease the risk of post-LP headache.[9] Slowly remove the needle in a fluid motion. One may apply a band-aid or gauze with tape over the needle insertion site. Traditionally, the patient is instructed to lie flat for 30 minutes following the procedure; however, one large meta-analysis found no difference in post-LP headache with bedrest versus early mobilization.[10]

3.7 Complications

- Post-LP (spinal) headache
- CSF leak
- Infection/Meningitis
- Downward herniation
- Spinal epidural hematoma
- Nerve root injury
- Intracranial subdural hematoma
- Epidermoid cyst

3.8 Expert Suggestions/Troubleshooting

With the patient lying a few inches from the edge of the bed, placing a large sterile sheet that covers the edge of the bed allows the operator to use the bed as a sterile shelf to hold instruments.

If the patient experiences sharp radiating pain down the leg, this suggests the needle has contacted a spinal nerve root. The operator should back the needle out to the deep dermal layer and aim a new trajectory opposite the side on which the patient experienced pain. For example, if a patient experiences sharp pain radiating down the right leg, the trajectory should be adjusted to aim more toward the patient's left side.

If the operator has clearly palpated the lamina with the needle tip and is confident in having passed through the interlaminar space and ligamentum flavum, and is again encountering bone without CSF flow, it is likely the needle is resting on the posterior aspect of the vertebral body. With the stylet in place, withdraw the needle a centimeter and check for CSF egress. If there is still no CSF flow, pull the needle back to the dermal layer and try a new trajectory.

If at any point during the procedure, the patient is complaining of excruciating pain and cannot tolerate the procedure, the operator must determine whether the patient requires additional medication or if the procedure should be aborted. At times, it is prudent to avoid moderate sedation and instead perform the LP under direct fluoroscopic guidance.

In a patient with a history of lumbar spine surgery, one should obtain imaging of the lumbar spine prior to the LP to evaluate the lumbar anatomy. One should understand the relevant anatomy prior to performing the LP. For example, one would not expect to palpate a spinous process or lamina in a patient with a history of lumbar laminectomy. A patient with a history of spinal fusion surgery may have a solid bony fusion mass that precludes the passage of the spinal needle into the lumbar cistern via a traditional LP trajectory. This can best be evaluated with a CT of the lumbar spine. In such cases, it would be prudent to perform the LP under fluoroscopic guidance if access to the lumbar cistern is still thought to be feasible based upon imaging or search for an alternative means of CSF access.

In a patient with challenging anatomy, a paramedian entry point may be used, thereby bypassing the supraspinous and interspinous ligaments, and instead traversing the paraspinal muscles. This is especially helpful in older patients with hypertrophied spinous processes or calcified ligaments.

References

[1] Czosnyka M, Czosnyka Z, Momjian S, Pickard JD. Cerebrospinal fluid dynamics. Physiol Meas. 2004; 25(5):R51–R76

[2] Sakka L, Coll G, Chazal J. Anatomy and physiology of cerebrospinal fluid. Eur Ann Otorhinolaryngol Head Neck Dis. 2011; 128(6):309–316

[3] Soleiman J, Demaerel P, Rocher S, Maes F, Marchal G. Magnetic resonance imaging study of the level of termination of the conus medullaris and the thecal sac: influence of age and gender. Spine. 2005; 30(16):1875–1880

[4] van Crevel H, Hijdra A, de Gans J. Lumbar puncture and the risk of herniation: when should we first perform CT? J Neurol. 2002; 249(2):129–137

[5] Brown MW, Yilmaz TS, Kasper EM. Iatrogenic spinal hematoma as a complication of lumbar puncture: what is the risk and best management plan? Surg Neurol Int. 2016; 7 Suppl 22:S581–S589

[6] Domenicucci M, Mancarella C, Santoro G, et al. Spinal epidural hematomas: personal experience and literature review of more than 1000 cases. J Neurosurg Spine. 2017; 27(2):198–208

[7] Williams J, Lye DCB, Umapathi T. Diagnostic lumbar puncture: minimizing complications. Intern Med J. 2008; 38(7):587–591

[8] Richman JM, Joe EM, Cohen SR, et al. Bevel direction and postdural puncture headache: a meta-analysis. Neurologist. 2006; 12(4):224–228

[9] Strupp M, Brandt T, Müller A. Incidence of post-lumbar puncture syndrome reduced by reinserting the stylet: a randomized prospective study of 600 patients. J Neurol. 1998; 245(9):589–592

[10] Thoennissen J, Herkner H, Lang W, Domanovits H, Laggner AN, Müllner M. Does bed rest after cervical or lumbar puncture prevent headache? A systematic review and meta-analysis. CMAJ. 2001; 165(10):1311–1316

4 Lumbar Drain

Neil Majmundar, Gurkirat Kohli, R. Nick Hernandez, and Rachid Assina

Abstract

Lumbar drain placement is a procedure performed at the bedside or in the operating room to allow for controlled drainage of cerebrospinal fluid (CSF). This chapter will review the relevant anatomy, indications, contraindications, equipment, technique, complications, and suggestions for placement of lumbar drains.

Keywords: lumbar drain, cerebrospinal fluid, hydrocephalus, CSF leak, CSF diversion

4.1 Introduction

A lumbar drain (LD) is a catheter that is inserted into the lumbar subarachnoid space to provide continuous access for cerebrospinal fluid (CSF) drainage. This is a sterile procedure that can be performed both at the bedside or in the operating room. Once the LD catheter is inserted into the thecal sac, it is then connected to a collection system which is used to collect CSF and monitor the output in a precise and controlled manner. A transducer can also be connected to the tubing to allow monitoring of intrathecal pressure, although the drain is not generally used for this purpose. In this chapter, we discuss the relevant anatomy, indications and contraindications, equipment, technique, troubleshooting if the drain malfunctions, and related complications.

4.2 Relevant Anatomy/Physiology

The choroid plexus, located throughout the intracranial ventricular system, produces the majority of CSF circulating within the central nervous system (CNS). At any point, there is approximately 125 to 150 mL of CSF circulating in adults with approximately 20% of the total CSF being located in the ventricles. The rest of the CSF is present in the subarachnoid cisterns. CSF flows from the lateral ventricles into the third ventricle via the foramen of Monro. From the third ventricle, CSF travels through the aqueduct of Sylvius into the fourth ventricle. It then exits the fourth ventricle medially through the foramen of Magendie, or laterally through the foramina of Luschka to circulate around the brain and spinal cord in the subarachnoid space. CSF is then reabsorbed into the venous circulation by the superior sagittal sinus through the arachnoid granulations projecting into the subarachnoid space. CSF is replaced approximately three to four times a day with approximately 400 to 500 mL produced per day.

In adults, the conus medullaris which marks the end of the spinal cord is usually located at the L1 or L2 vertebral levels. The subarachnoid space continues to the S2 vertebral level. The lumbar cistern is the enlargement of the subarachnoid space between the conus medullaris of the spinal cord and the end of the dura mater at the S2 vertebral level. The lumbar cistern, the site for performing the lumbar puncture, contains the lumbosacral nerve roots forming the cauda equina, the filum terminale, and cerebrospinal fluid.

4.3 Indications

4.3.1 Craniotomy

Lumbar drains are used to facilitate brain relaxation in cases for which significant brain retraction is expected to decrease postoperative cerebral edema. These cases include anterior skull base cases, retrosigmoid approaches, far lateral approaches, and suboccipital craniectomies, amongst others.[1,2] In these cases, the drain is generally placed preoperatively and clamped. During the procedure, if additional relaxation is required, the drain can be opened to drain the desired amount of CSF. The LD can then either remain in place postoperatively, or be removed at the end of the case.

4.3.2 Endoscopic Skull Base Surgery

Lumbar drains are commonly used in endoscopic skull base surgeries. These cases have a high rate of CSF leak because the dural defect is situated in a dependent location. An LD may be placed prior to or after an endoscopic endonasal approach to reduce intracranial pressure (ICP) to allow for the skull base defect to heal and prevent postoperative CSF leak.[3] The LD generally remains in place for a few days during the postoperative period, draining the desired amount each hour or every other hour, until satisfactory dural closure is suspected and the patient does not have any CSF leak.

4.3.3 CSF Leak

In cases of spontaneous or traumatic CSF leak, an LD can be placed prior to the attempted closure. This includes cases of CSF rhinorrhea, otorrhea, and spinal leaks. An added benefit of preoperative placement is the ability to administer intrathecal fluorescein.[4] The LD can then either be removed after performing the repair or be left in place during the postoperative period to facilitate dural closure. Placement of the LD significantly improves the rate of closure and limits the potential complications following a persistent CSF leak.

4.3.4 Normal Pressure Hydrocephalus

Patients who are being diagnosed with normal pressure hydrocephalus (NPH) can undergo LD placement as part of the workup.[5] If NPH is suspected based upon patient history, examination, and imaging findings, the patient is admitted and an LD is placed. Prior to placement, the patient is evaluated by physical therapy (PT). After drain placement, the desired amount of CSF is drained each day, and the patient undergoes daily PT evaluations to see if gait, balance, and gait speed improve. During LD placement, opening pressure can also be checked and CSF can be collected for analysis to confirm that the correct diagnosis is being made. If the patient improves clinically after LD placement, permanent CSF diversion with a ventriculoperitoneal or lumboperitoneal shunt is recommended.[6]

4.3.5 Thoracoabdominal Aortic Surgery

Lumbar drains can also be placed for thoracoabdominal aortic surgery. Stenting or repair of the aorta can alter blood flow through important segmental arteries. LD placement allows for CSF diversion and thereby reduce pressure in the intrathecal space. This may increase spinal cord perfusion pressure and result in the reduction of ischemic injury to the spinal cord.[7]

4.3.6 Miscellaneous

Lumbar drains can also be placed for a variety of other reasons. If a patient requires repeat sampling of CSF or repeat drainage in cases of communicating hydrocephalus, an LD can be placed. An LD can also be placed in cases of CSF leak following spine surgery.

4.4 Contraindications

The contraindications to the insertion of an LD include the following.

4.4.1 Intracranial Mass Lesion

A potential complication with placement of an LD is cerebral herniation, which can lead to compression of integral neurovascular structures and result in mortality.[8] Neuroimaging, either computed tomography (CT) or magnetic resonance imaging (MRI), is important to identify any pathology such as hematomas, hemorrhages, masses, and abscesses that can potentially increase the ICP resulting in shifting of the brain. Insertion of an LD can further exacerbate the brain herniation in cases of existing increased ICP by reducing the pressure within the spinal compartment.

4.4.2 Obstructive Hydrocephalus

Any obstruction of normal CSF flow can increase ICP, placing the patient at risk of cerebral herniation. Placement of an LD can increase the pressure gradient between the cranial and the spinal compartments leading to further herniation.

4.4.3 Skin Infection/Spinal Epidural Abscess

Placement of an LD should be avoided in patients with clinical findings and imaging suggesting of a presence of an epidural abscess. Insertion of the needle directly through the abscess increases the risk of meningitis and subdural infection. LD should also be avoided in the presence of any superficial skin infection over the lumbar region to avoid risking further spread of the infection into deeper tissues with the needle.

4.4.4 Coagulopathy/Thrombocytopenia/ Anticoagulant Therapy

As with a lumbar puncture, patients with bleeding disorders or currently on antiplatelet or anticoagulant therapy have an increased risk of developing a spinal epidural hematoma.[9]

4.5 Equipment

- Sterile prep kit
- Local anesthetic
- Sterile gown, gloves, and face mask
- LD kit (▶ Fig. 4.1)
  ○ 14-gauge Tuohy needle
  ○ Drainage catheter (▶ Fig. 4.2) with guidewire
  ○ Collection system
- Dressing

4.6 Technique

4.6.1 Positioning and Equipment Setup

Prior to the start of the procedure, the patient's imaging should be reviewed, including any relevant cranial and spinal imaging. A single dose of antibiotics may be given prior to the procedure.

The patient should be positioned in the lateral decubitus position with chin to the chest and the legs flexed to the abdomen, thereby increasing the interlaminar distance. The iliac crest should be palpated to aim for insertion at

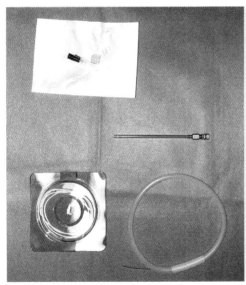

Fig. 4.1 Lumbar drain (LD) kit: Caps for the catheter once inserted (*top*), 14-guage Tuohy needle (*middle*), LD catheter (*bottom left*), and LD catheter guidewire (*bottom right*).

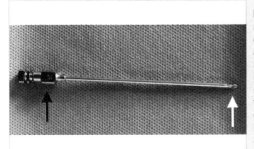

Fig. 4.2 Lumbar drain Tuohy needle. Black arrow shows the gauge (14), and the white arrow points to the bevel. The needle should be inserted with both of these facing up (to minimize risk of nerve root transection) and turned 90 degrees (to direct the catheter rostrally) once the thecal sac is accessed.

the L4–L5 or L3–L4 interspace. This should be marked out, as depicted in ▶ Fig. 4.3.

The procedure site should then be prepped and draped in a sterile fashion.

Next, a local anesthetic should be administered superficially and then deep to provide adequate anesthesia during needle insertion.

After injecting the local anesthetic, the kit should be prepared. First, the 14-gauge Tuohy needle and its stylet should be checked. Next, the guidewire and catheter should be placed in a basin filled with sterile saline or water to ensure easy removal of the guidewire from the catheter during a later step. Once the catheter and guidewire have been placed in the basin, the wire can then be

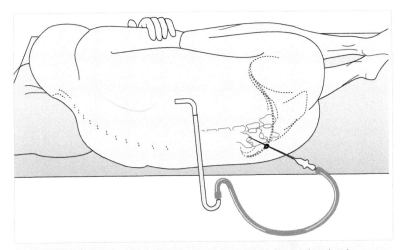

Fig. 4.3 Left lateral decubitus positioning for drain insertion. (Reproduced with permission from Mattle H, Mumenthaler M, Taub E, eds. Fundamentals of Neurology: An Illustrated Guide. 2nd Edition. Thieme; 2017.)

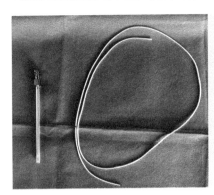

Fig. 4.4 14-guage Tuohy needle and the lumbar drain (LD) catheter with guidewire inserted.

inserted into the catheter. The collection system should be flushed proximally and distally to prevent air-locking of tubing.

4.6.2 Procedure

Once adequate local anesthesia is confirmed by palpating the entry site, the procedure may commence. With the bevel facing upwards (number upwards on most kits), insert the Touhy needle (▶ Fig. 4.4). Slowly advance the needle a few millimeters at a time, while concurrently processing the tactile feedback from the needle. The needle will advance through the skin and subcutaneous tissue. If a midline approach is chosen, the next structures are the supraspinous ligament, interspinous ligament, and then lamina if the needle is a few millimeters above or below the interlaminar space. The needle can then be worked up or down the lamina until the interlaminar space is encountered. The needle will then traverse the ligamentum flavum, epidural space, and dura before entering the subarachnoid space. There is a "give" in resistance once the needle traverses the ligamentum flavum.

At any point during the procedure if the needle is thought to be in the subarachnoid space, the stylet can be removed to check for CSF. Once CSF flow is confirmed, the bevel of the needle should then be turned toward the head to allow insertion of the catheter. In most systems, the needle is turned so that the number is facing toward the head of the patient. It is important to leave the stylet in place while reaching for the catheter to prevent excessive CSF drainage. Once the catheter is ready, the stylet is removed and the catheter is inserted to the 15-cm mark at the skin. If at any point resistance is encountered, the catheter should not be forced. The needle angle can be adjusted, and the catheter insertion can be continued if this solves the problem. At no point should the needle be advanced during the placement of the catheter nor should the catheter be pulled back out of the needle once advanced without pulling the needle out with the catheter, as this can result in shearing of the catheter. The wire must also not be removed prior to removal of the Tuohy needle as this can also damage the catheter.

Once the catheter is advanced to 15 cm at the skin, the Tuohy needle is removed from over the catheter. During this step, secure the catheter in place with one hand making sure that it is not displaced. Next, remove the guidewire from within the catheter, again ensuring that the catheter remains in its proper position at the skin.

The catheter can then be connected to the collection system with the catheter cap included in the kit. During cap placement, it is important to ensure that the end of catheter is not torn. A silk tie can be used to secure the catheter tip to the cap. The catheter can then be connected to the collection system.

The drapes can then be removed and the catheter can be secured to the patient's skin with clear adhesive dressings.

4.7 Complications

4.7.1 Headache

CSF leak causes intrathecal hypotension resulting in traction on the meninges and cranial nerves. If the patient experiences significant headaches following drainage, the amount of CSF drained can be reduced or drainage can be stopped as this may indicate significant intracranial hypotension.

4.7.2 Cerebral Herniation

Overdrainage of CSF can result in downward herniation. In this case, the patient should immediately be placed in a Trendelenburg position and drainage must be stopped immediately.

4.7.3 Infection

There is a risk of meningitis, cellulitis, and ventriculitis due to poor sterile technique during insertion or prolonged use of the drain. The risk of meningitis has been reported at 4% and most often is a result of infection from skin flora. Prophylactic antibiotics can be given to cover for gram positive organisms such as first-generation cephalosporins, although there is a lack of evidence that this is protective against meningitis.[10] Infections are best prevented by following strict sterile techniques during placement and removing the drain as soon as possible.

4.7.4 Retained Catheter

This is a concerning complication of LD placement and can occur anywhere along the tract of the drain due to shearing of the catheter from the needle. This is best avoided by not pulling the catheter while the catheter is still within the needle. It is also critical to remove the needle prior to the guidewire.

4.7.5 Spinal Cord Injury/Parethesia

The needle may penetrate the nerve roots leading to paresthesia, extremity weakness, or pain. If the patient reports these symptoms, an attempt can be made to place the drain at a different interspinous space. These symptoms are usually temporary as damage to nerve roots is not typically permanent. Damage to the cord can be prevented by correctly using surface landmarks to identify a safe site for insertion.

4.8 Expert Suggestions/Troubleshooting

4.8.1 Overdrainage

The large diameter of the needle can result in excessive loss of CSF. The needle should be covered with the thumb quickly after the stylet is removed and the catheter should also be closed with the connector. If the patient shows any signs or symptoms of overdrainage during CSF drainage, it must be stopped immediately. If the catheter has been draining, and the patient develops symptoms of headache or has a change in neurological examination, the drain should be clamped immediately. The patient's bed should be placed in Trendelenburg position, and head should be lowered.

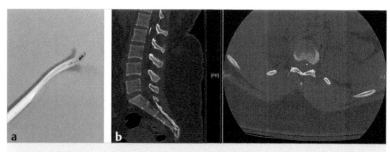

Fig. 4.5 **(a)** The removed portion of a sheared catheter. The remaining catheter was all intradural in this particular patient and was not removed. **(b)** Computed tomography (CT) scan showing sagittal and axial views of the retained intradural catheter.

4.8.2 Catheter Shearing

The catheter should not be pulled through the needle once it has been placed to avoid shearing of the catheter over the needle. Once the catheter has been inserted, the needle should not be advanced. The guidewire should also not be removed from the catheter before the needle is removed to prevent shearing. In certain cases, one may not realize that the catheter had been sheared during placement until the catheter has been removed. This results in snapping of the catheter during removal, and the complication of a retained catheter (▶ Fig. 4.5). If the retained catheter is fully intradural, we do not recommend removal unless the patient is symptomatic. If the catheter is both intra- and extradural, the catheter must be removed. If the catheter is extradural, in most cases removal is not warranted.

4.8.3 No CSF Egress

During placement of the drain, if there is no egress of CSF after multiple attempts either a new level can be attempted, or imaging can be obtained to evaluate for any aberrant anatomy. In addition, the drain can be attempted to be placed under fluoroscopic guidance. It may be that the needle has entered the lumbar cistern, but the catheter cannot be passed. In certain cases, the needle can be slightly pulled back or can be repositioned so that the tip of the needle is pointing more rostrally while the head of the needle (and the hand) is dropped.

4.8.4 Severe Pre-existing CSF Leak

Insertion of an LD is particularly challenging in patients with extant CSF leak, resulting in low CSF volume within the thecal sac. In such cases, it may be helpful to place the patient steeply in reverse Trendelenburg position and/or to utilize fluoroscopy. Occasionally, in patients with minimal remaining CSF within the thecal sac, it is possible to situate the drain within the subarachnoid space without any return of CSF. When this is suspected, iodinated contrast can be administered through the drain to establish whether it is appropriately placed.

4.9 Conclusion

Lumbar drains, while a seemingly simple procedure, play an important role in the treatment of several neurological pathologies. This chapter has highlighted some of the indications, techniques, and complications encountered.

References

[1] Ackerman PD, Spencer DA, Prabhu VC. The efficacy and safety of preoperative lumbar drain placement in anterior skull base surgery. J Neurol Surg Rep. 2013; 74(1):1–9

[2] Bien AG, Bowdino B, Moore G, Leibrock L. Utilization of preoperative cerebrospinal fluid drain in skull base surgery. Skull Base. 2007; 17(2):133–139

[3] Zwagerman NT, Shin S, Wang EW, Fernandez-Miranda JC, Synderman CH, Gardner PA. A prospective, randomized control trial for lumbar drain placement after endoscopic endonasal skull base surgery. J Neurol Surg B Skull Base. 2016; 77(S 02):LFP-13–03

[4] Stokken J, Recinos PF, Woodard T, Sindwani R. The utility of lumbar drains in modern endoscopic skull base surgery. Curr Opin Otolaryngol Head Neck Surg. 2015; 23(1):78–82

[5] Woodworth GF, McGirt MJ, Williams MA, Rigamonti D. Cerebrospinal fluid drainage and dynamics in the diagnosis of normal pressure hydrocephalus. Neurosurgery. 2009; 64(5):919–925, discussion 925–926

[6] Chotai S, Medel R, Herial NA, Medhkour A. External lumbar drain: a pragmatic test for prediction of shunt outcomes in idiopathic normal pressure hydrocephalus. Surg Neurol Int. 2014; 5:12

[7] Fedorow CA, Moon MC, Mutch WA, Grocott HP. Lumbar cerebrospinal fluid drainage for thoracoabdominal aortic surgery: rationale and practical considerations for management. Anesth Analg. 2010; 111(1):46–58

[8] Wang K, Liu Z, Chen X, Lou M, Yin J. Clinical characteristics and outcomes of patients with cerebral herniation during continuous lumbar drainage. Turk Neurosurg. 2013; 23(5):653–657

[9] Sladky JH, Piwinski SE. Lumbar puncture technique and lumbar drains. Atlas Oral Maxillofac Surg Clin North Am. 2015; 23(2):169–176

[10] Coplin WM, Avellino AM, Kim DK, Winn HR, Grady MS. Bacterial meningitis associated with lumbar drains: a retrospective cohort study. J Neurol Neurosurg Psychiatry. 1999; 67(4):468–473

5 Parenchymal Intracranial Pressure Monitor

Abstract

Intracranial pressure (ICP) monitors are a common and useful tool in the Neuro-ICU. Here, the following topics related to insertion of an ICP monitor are discussed in detail: relevant anatomy and physiology, indications/contraindications, equipment, technique, complications, and expert suggestions.

Keywords: ICP monitor, traumatic brain injury, CPP intracranial pressure

5.1 Introduction

An intracranial pressure (ICP) monitor is any device that is utilized to measure ICP. This can be done by direct measurement of the epidural, subdural, intra-parenchymal, or intraventricular pressure. The intraparenchymal monitor is the most common device utilized for this purpose and its application will be described in this chapter.

Several intraparenchymal ICP monitor devices are commercially available. The Camino (Natus, Pleasanton, CA, USA) and the Codman Microsensor (DePuy Synthes, West Chester, PA, USA) are two of the more widely used devices. The Camino probe contains a fiber-optic transducer whereas the Microsensor uses a strain gauge to detect electrical conductance. Specific procedural steps described below are most closely applicable to the Camino (Natus, Pleasanton, CA, USA) device.

All ICP monitor systems provide instantaneous measurement of pressure, graphic display of the pressure waveform, and a record of ICP trends over time. This data is typically displayed in mm Hg and is used to guide management of elevated ICP in the setting of trauma, neoplasm, craniosynostosis, liver failure, and idiopathic intracranial hypertension. ▶ Fig. 5.1 demonstrates a schematic representing an ICP monitor setup.

5.2 Relevant Anatomy and Physiology

The intracranial cavity is occupied by three substances, the brain parenchyma, cerebrospinal fluid (CSF), and blood volume. According to the Monro-Kellie Doctrine, expansion of one of these substances must be balanced by reduction in another to maintain a consistent pressure in a closed cranial cavity.[1] When expansion of one of these substances surpasses what can be effectively

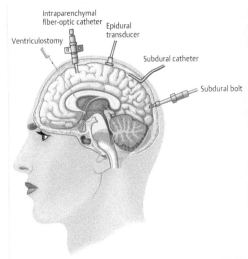

Intraparenchymal fiber-optic catheter

Epidural transducer

Ventriculostomy

Subdural catheter

Subdural bolt

Fig. 5.1 Schematic of intracranial pressure (ICP) monitor.

displaced by the other two substances, then an increase in ICP occurs. The brain parenchyma exists throughout the cranial cavity. CSF is elaborated by the choroid plexus flows from the lateral ventricles, through the foramen of Monro, into the third ventricle, through the Sylvian aqueduct, into the fourth ventricle, through the foramina of Luschka and Magendie, and into the subarachnoid cisternal spaces around the brain, spinal cord, and spinal nerves. The CSF is reabsorbed from the subarachnoid space into the superior sagittal sinus. The blood exists in the vascular space occupied by the arteries, capillaries, veins, and sinuses. The interdependent relationship of these spaces in a closed cavity creates a continuity of pressure throughout the closed system. With a few notable exceptions in the setting of trapped ventricles, hemispheres, obstructive pathology, and the posterior fossa, the measurement of ICP at one location in the cranial vault can be assumed to represent the pressure throughout the intracranial space. ▶ Fig. 5.2 depicts the Monro-Kellie Doctrine.

5.3 Indications

Disease states in which ICP monitoring may be beneficial include, but are not limited to, trauma, neoplasm, craniosynostosis, liver failure, anoxic injury, and idiopathic intracranial hypertension. By far the most common indication for ICP monitor placement is traumatic brain injury (TBI).

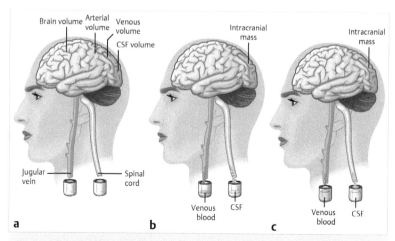

Fig. 5.2 Monro-Kellie Doctrine. **(a)** Normal cranial cavity. **(b)** Small intracranial mass causing displacement of venous blood and cerebrospinal fluid (CSF). **(c)** Large intracranial mass causing greater displacement of venous blood and CSF.

5.3.1 Recommendations from the 4th Edition Brain Trauma Foundation Guidelines[2]

Level I or IIA

There was insufficient evidence to support a level I or IIA recommendation for ICP monitoring.

Level IIB

Management of severe TBI patients using information from ICP monitoring is recommended to reduce in-hospital and 2-week postinjury mortality.

5.3.2 Recommendations from the Prior (3rd) Edition Not Supported by Evidence Meeting Current Standards

- ICP should be monitored in all salvageable patients with a severe TBI (GCS 3–8 after resuscitation) and an abnormal computed tomography (CT) scan. An abnormal CT scan of the head is one that reveals hematomas, contusions, swelling, herniation, or compressed basal cisterns.
- ICP monitoring is indicated in patients with severe TBI with a normal CT scan if two or more of the following features are noted at admission: age over 40 years, unilateral or bilateral motor posturing, and systolic blood pressure (BP) < 90 mm Hg.

5.4 Contraindications

The following are relative contraindications to insertion of an ICP monitor:

- Coagulopathy
- Thrombocytopenia
- Recent antiplatelet therapy
- Uremic platelet dysfunction
- Recent thrombolytic therapy
- Mass lesion obstructing catheter trajectory
- Scalp infection
- Hydrocephalus (ventricular catheter placement is preferred)

5.5 Equipment

The majority of equipment needed for ICP monitor insertion is contained in a pre-packaged cranial access kit (see ▸ Fig. 5.3). Sometimes the cranial access kit and the ICP monitor fiber-optic catheter/drill bit will be in separate boxes. Below is a list of the necessary equipments:

- Fiber-optic catheter/Bolt (▸ Fig. 5.4)
  - Monitor
- Twist drill with appropriate drill bit for ICP monitor
  - Allen wrench for adjusting drill guard
- #15 blade scalpel
  - 18-gauge spinal needle
  - Obturator probe
  - Screw driver for calibrating fiber-optic catheter

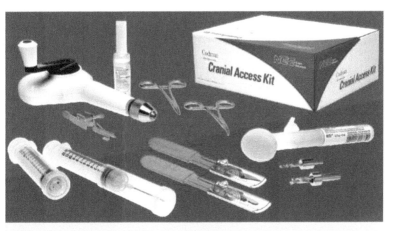

Fig. 5.3 Cranial access kit. Courtesy: Integra LifeSciences.

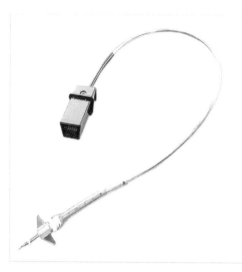

Fig. 5.4 Camino fiber-optic catheter, bolt, calibration module. Courtesy: Natus.

- Lidocaine with epinephrine
- Cap, mask, gown, sterile gloves (× 2), perforated sterile drape, and chuck
- Shaver, shaver head, alcohol or betadine skin prep, marking pen, ruler, and gauze
- 2–0 silk stitch (× 2)
- Sterile flush (× 2)
  ○ Adhesive dressing (× 3)
  ○ Petroleum dressing

5.6 Technique

5.6.1 Preparation

- Review CT scan to rule out any structural contraindication and evaluate planned trajectory.
- Review results of relevant laboratory studies.

5.6.2 Medications

- Oxygen should be administered via face mask if the patient is not intubated.
- Antibiotics with gram positive coverage are used for skin flora prophylaxis. Cefazolin is used most commonly. If using a cephalosporin, the medication should be administered as an intravenous (IV) push 5 minutes prior to incision. Administration of additional prophylactic antibiotics beyond this single peri-procedural dose is not recommended.

- Antihypertensive agents should be used to maintain the systolic blood pressure less than 140 mm Hg during and immediately after the procedure. The calcium channel blocker nicardipine is most commonly used due to rapid action and ease of titration. Nitroprusside should not be used as it will cause an increase in ICP.
- Sedation is usually accomplished with propofol, midazolam, and fentanyl all of which will confer additional antihypertensive effects.
- Lidocaine with or without epinephrine can be used for local anesthesia.

5.6.3 Positioning/Equipment Setup

- Position the patient supine with the head of the bed at 20 degrees. The patient's head should slightly overhang the top of bed. If there is a headboard on the bed it should be removed. The bed height should be adjusted for operator comfort.
- Shave the scalp widely.
- Wipe the shaved area of the scalp with alcohol.
- Dry the scalp and clearly mark the midline.
- Mark a point 3 cm behind the hairline on the midpupillary line.

5.6.4 Procedure

- Prep skin with chlorhexidine or betadine solution.
- Once skin is prepped, you may begin setting up sterile field with all the equipment.
- Inject local anesthetic with epinephrine to marked site.
- Make stab incision over marked site.
- Clear off periosteum.
- Set the drill guard based on the combined thickness of the scalp and skull as measured from the coronal CT recon. Usually, this is approximately 2 cm.
- Drill perpendicular to skull carefully, as this drill bit will easily penetrate the skull and risk of plunging is high.
- Once through the skull, verify with obturator probe by feeling for dura.
- Clear away any bony debris with a water syringe flush.
- Loosen the diaphragm cap at the top of the bolt and advance the obturator probe so that it protrudes out of the tip of the bolt by 1 cm. Re-tighten the diaphragm cap to hold the obturator probe in this position. The obturator probe will help guide the bolt into the burr hole.
- Begin to screw bolt in place.
- Once the threads of the bolt engage bone, loosen the diaphragm cap and remove the obturator probe.
- Continue screwing the bolt in until it is finger-tight.
- Insert long needle from kit into bolt to make small durotomy.

- Re-insert the obturator probe fully into the bolt, passing through the durotomy and into the brain to create a tract within the parenchyma.
- Leave the obturator probe in place while preparing to insert the monitor itself.
- For most devices, it is necessary to calibrate the ICP monitor by setting it to zero at atmospheric pressure. For the Camino ICP monitor (Natus, Pleasanton, CA, USA), this is accomplished by rotating a screw on the calibration module (held up by an assistant) until the value on the monitor is 0.
- Remove the obturator probe.
- Fiber-optic monitor insertion for Camino (Natus, Pleasanton, CA, USA):
  - Retract the fiber-optic wire within the plastic sleeve.
  - Snuggly couple the plastic sleeve to the diaphragm cap (cap should be loose).
  - Advance catheter 2 to 4 cm into brain parenchyma. (The red dot should lie within the clear part of the plastic sleeve.)
  - Tighten the diaphragm cap to secure the monitor.
- Plug into bedside ICP monitor, note pressure.
- Wrap with petroleum dressing.
- Secure catheter to sheath with adhesive dressing.

5.6.5 Postprocedure

- CT head to assess for appropriate placement of monitor and to rule out new hemorrhage.

5.7 Complications

5.7.1 Infection

Infection is a very rare complication of ICP monitor placement. In their review of 229 patients with ICP monitors, Guyot et al reported no incidence of infection.[3]

5.7.2 Hemorrhage

Gelabert-González et al have published the largest retrospective series to date of 1,000 patients with ICP monitors. Interestingly, in their study, of 87 patients with at least 1 abnormal coagulation parameter, 7 had a catheter-related hemorrhage (8%) compared with 18 hemorrhages among the 903 patients (2%) with normal coagulation parameters.[4] This highlights the importance of reviewing appropriate lab values prior to the procedure.

5.7.3 Motor Cortex Injury

Damage to the motor cortex can occur when a fiber-optic catheter is placed in an inappropriate posterior position. This complication can be avoided by ensuring that the burr hole site is at least 3 cm anterior to the coronal suture.

5.7.4 Superior Sagittal Sinus Injury

Injury to the superior sagittal sinus results from medial placement of an ICP monitor. This potentially fatal complication can be avoided by carefully marking the midline, selecting a burr hole site at least 2.5 cm lateral to the midline, and holding the twist drill firmly to avoid migration of the drill tip while beginning the burr hole.

5.8 Expert Suggestions/Troubleshooting

5.8.1 Scalp Bleeding

Excessive scalp bleeding can pose a challenge since most ICP monitors are placed outside of the operating room without readily available electrocautery. The risk of transecting a scalp artery can be minimized by using a small stab incision. Injecting local anesthetic with epinephrine will result in vasoconstriction. This is especially helpful if injected several minutes prior to incision. When bleeding from a scalp artery cannot be stopped with manual compression, a stitch can be thrown adjacent to the incision (on the lateral side where the blood supply originates) to tie off the bleeding vessel.

5.8.2 Entry Site

Most commonly, ICP monitors are placed on the right side. If there is small mass lesion including hematoma or contusion on any side that would likely be the side of hemicraniectomy in the setting of elevated ICP, it would be wise to place the ICP monitor on the contralateral side. If there is a possibility that CSF diversion is an option for management of ICP (larger than average ventricles) when medical treatment fails, it may be valuable to place the ICP monitor at Kocher's point upfront so that the fiber-optic catheter can be exchanged for an external ventricular drain in the future, should the clinical situation call for it, without having to plan and remark incisions.

5.8.3 Aberrant ICP Measurement

Immediately following ICP monitoring insertion, it is common for measurements to be falsely elevated. This should correct on its own and the ICP reading can be observed decreasing to an accurate measurement over several minutes.

A more intractable measurement problem occurs when the lead is inserted too deep. This results in tension on the lead, generating a falsely elevated ICP measurement. Using the obturator to create a tract within the parenchyma will mitigate the risk of this from occurring. Additionally, it may be useful to insert the monitor lead to target depth and then immediately pull back 2 mm to avoid "spring-loading" the lead.

Unexpected ICP changes later on may indicate lead displacement. It is very useful to take note of the exact position of the lead within the plastic sleeve (i.e., where the red dot is located). Any sudden ICP changes not consistent with the clinical scenario should prompt a thorough evaluation of the device, including removal of the dressing to confirm that the bolt is still secured appropriately in the skull and that the plastic sleeve and monitor lead are secured and correctly positioned relative to the bolt.

References

[1] Mokri B. The Monro-Kellie hypothesis: applications in CSF volume depletion. Neurology. 2001; 56(12):1746–1748

[2] Carney N, Totten AM, O'Reilly C, et al. Guidelines for the management of severe traumatic brain injury, fourth edition. Neurosurgery. 2017; 80(1):6–15

[3] Guyot LL, Dowling C, Diaz FG, Michael DB. Cerebral monitoring devices: analysis of complications. Acta Neurochir Suppl (Wien). 1998; 71:47–49

[4] Gelabert-González M, Ginesta-Galan V, Sernamito-García R, Allut AG, Bandin-Diéguez J, Rumbo RM. The Camino intracranial pressure device in clinical practice: assessment in a 1000 cases. Acta Neurochir (Wien). 2006; 148(4):435–441

6 Brain Tissue Oxygenation: Procedural Steps and Clinical Utility

Nitesh V. Patel, Matthew S. Parr, and John Kauffmann

Abstract

Cerebral oximetry ($PbtO_2$ monitoring) is the direct measurement of the partial pressure of oxygen within brain parenchyma. This chapter reviews the physiologic rationale for intracranial oxygenation monitoring, summarizes the clinical evidence evaluating its effectiveness, and discusses the placement, troubleshooting, and evaluation of intracranial brain oxygenation monitors.

Keywords: brain tissue oxygenation, intracranial monitoring, traumatic brain injury

6.1 Introduction

Following a neurologic insult, secondary brain injury may occur despite normal intracranial pressure (ICP) and normal cerebral perfusion pressure.[1] The goal of $PbtO_2$ monitoring is to directly assess the metabolic state of the injured brain to determine if treatment is needed to improve cerebral blood flow and oxygenation. In states of generalized brain injury, measurements of mean arterial pressure (MAP), ICP, and resultant cerebral perfusion pressure (CPP) become important guiding points for therapy. However, augmentation of MAP to maintain adequate CPP comes with systemic risks. Since the overarching goal of maintaining appropriate CPP is to provide sufficient blood flow to meet the metabolic demands of the brain, instead of simply measuring ICP and augmenting CPP, direct measurement of brain tissue oxygenation theoretically could be a more useful guiding parameter.

6.2 Relevant Anatomy and Physiology

6.2.1 Anatomic Considerations

Monitor placement requires opening the calvaria and meninges. Optimally, an area of cortex that is relatively noneloquent and easy to access is the target. The frontal lobes, anterior to the coronal suture, are an ideal place for intracranial monitors. Choosing a point in the midpupillary line, approximately 2 to 3 cm behind the hairline, serves as a good start. If the patient's hairline is not clear, palpation of the coronal suture should help guide entry site. Approximately 3 cm anterior to the coronal suture is usually a safe region.

6.2.2 Physiologic Principles

At rest, the brain accounts for 25% of the metabolic demand of the human body. Many observational studies have borne out that low $PbtO_2$ correlates with increased risk of death and poor outcome in traumatic brain injury. $PbtO_2$ values less than 20 mm Hg appear to be harmful.[2,3,4,5,6,7] Despite the well-established correlation between low $PbtO_2$ and adverse outcome, it is unclear whether $PbtO_2$ goal-directed treatment protocols can alter the disease course of traumatic brain injury. There have been a handful of cohort studies comparing treatment protocols for traumatic brain injury based upon monitoring of ICP in conjunction with $PbtO_2$ versus monitoring of ICP in isolation. The results of these have been mixed. Several studies have shown that $PbtO_2$ monitoring improved outcomes.[8][9] One study demonstrated that outcomes were better in the ICP monitoring group without $PbtO_2$ monitoring,[10] and others have shown no difference.[11,12]

6.2.3 Devices

A number of $PbtO_2$ monitoring devices are commercially available, including the Licox (Integra, Plainsboro, NJ, USA), the Neurovent (Raumedic AG, Münchberg, Germany), and the Oxylab (Oxford Optronix Ltd, Oxford, UK). For all such devices, a twist drill is used to facilitate insertion of a probe into the white matter of the brain. The Licox probe contains a Clark polarographic electrode composed of a silver electrode (anode) and a platinum electrode (cathode) with a membranous covering. As oxygen enters, it is reduced at the cathode and the anode-to-cathode electron flow results in production of water. The rate at which this reaction occurs is directly proportional to the amount of oxygen present; more oxygen means more reduction and more electron inclusion. This creates a Galvanic current (direct current) and can be converted into a partial oxygen pressure. The Neurovent and Oxylab probes contain luminescent ruthenium which emits light. The ruthenium luminophore is deactivated by oxygen. This process is known as luminescence quenching. A photodetector measures the amount of light emitted which can then be used to calculate the $PbtO_2$[13] (see ► Fig. 6.1). Both methods are highly reliable and accurate. Response time and precision tend to be slightly better in the optical luminescent model; however, clinical significance is negligible. There is concern for drift as with any intracranial monitoring device, that is, unintended change in calibration over time. The basic components of each of these devices consist: (1) fiber-optic or electrical lead/wire, (2) anchoring bolt for cranial securement, and (3) external monitor to which the lead/wire connects.

6.3 Indications

Theoretically, $PbtO_2$ monitoring can be a powerful tool in the management of patients with suspected compromise of cerebral perfusion. At the present time,

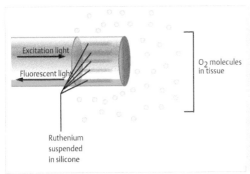

Fig. 6.1 Optical luminescent PtO$_2$ monitor. Oxygen molecules in tissue interact with the ruthenium in the lead. A light source drives a beam of light into the system which then interacts with the oxygen modified ruthenium and the wavelength of this light changes. This change is detected by the monitoring system and converted to a PbtO$_2$ value.

there is no high-quality evidence demonstrating that treatment algorithms based upon PbtO$_2$ measurements improve clinical outcomes. PbtO$_2$ monitoring is employed most frequently in the setting of traumatic brain injury. The optimal insertion site for a PbtO$_2$ monitor is unknown. To obtain a global assessment of brain oxygenation, it may be placed in the frontal white matter contralateral to the injury. Alternatively, the "penumbral" brain tissue surrounding the site of maximal injury may be a logical site for the device to be inserted. Currently, there is no evidence to support one approach over the other.

In clinical practice, PbtO$_2$ monitoring is believed to offer particular benefit in poly-trauma patients with both brain and lung injuries. In such cases, PbtO$_2$ measurement can help to determine an appropriate balance between neurologic and pulmonary protective treatments.

Another possible application for PbtO$_2$ monitoring is the detection of vasospasm in subarachnoid hemorrhage. While theoretically promising, a prospective observational study concluded that ischemic events detected by this method could not be corrected rapidly enough to improve outcomes.[14]

6.4 Contraindications

The use of invasive PtO$_2$ monitoring is contraindicated in patients who are at substantial risk of complications that would outweigh the clinical benefit of the real-time oxygenation data. This includes patients with an increased risk of hemorrhage, as well as those with infection of the tissue into which the device will be inserted. Magnetic resonance imaging (MRI) compatibility is device-dependent, and certain devices may be contraindicated in an MRI environment.

6.5 Equipment

6.5.1 Pre-Op Checklist and Equipment/Supplies

• Nursing staff and assistant if available
• Semi-sterile room
• Drapes
• Personal protective equipment (PPE) including gown, gloves, mask, and hat
• Extra packages of sterile gauze, saline, and dressing supplies
• Review of patient's imaging and blood work
• Intracranial access supplies and PbtO$_2$ monitor supplies (usually part of kit)
• Ensure all team members know the key procedural steps and know where additional supplies are in case replacements are needed

6.5.2 Sedation

In most patients requiring ICP and/or oxygenation monitoring, intubation may already have been performed. However, in some instances, patients may be protecting their own airway. In intubated patients, intravenous sedatives such as propofol, fentanyl, ketamine, or midazolam may be used. These sedatives may be used in a number of combinations depending on the specific needs of the patient. Factors to consider are blood pressure, mental status, clinical examination, and known cardiac issues. It may be helpful to have an anesthesiology team member immediately available.

6.6 Technique

6.6.1 Positioning

Positioning for PtO$_2$ monitors is similar to that for placement of a typical ICP monitor or an external ventricular drain. The patient is positioned supine with the head of the bed raised to approximately 30 degrees. An absorbent pad is placed under the scalp and care is taken to ensure positioning will not facilitate easy head rotation. The side of the scalp to be incised should be clearly accessible and obstructions such as intravenous lines, cables, and other equipment should be moved. The height of the bed should be comfortable for the operator and the area around the bed should be kept clear to facilitate easy movement and access to the supply table.

6.6.2 Incision Planning

In cases where there is bilateral or diffuse cerebral edema, the nondominant side is preferred—if damage occurs, it will have less impact on outcome. Along

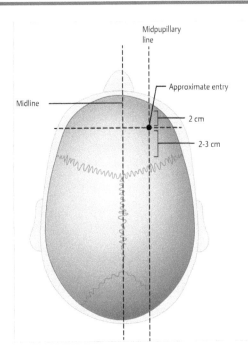

Midpupillary line

Approximate entry

Midline

2 cm

2-3 cm

Fig. 6.2 Entry incision. An entry is typically planned in the midpupillary line, approximately 2 cm behind the hairline or 2 to 3 cm in front of the coronal suture. It is important to mark the midline before planning the incision.

the midpupillary line and approximately 2 to 3 cm behind the hairline, a small stab incision is planned (▶ Fig. 6.2).

6.6.3 Prep and Drape

The surgical site is shaved of any hair in the region and care is taken to ensure enough hair is removed such that a dressing will stick well to the skin in the area. The area is cleaned with alcohol and then is re-marked. Next, the area is prepped using either a standard iodine based wound prep kit or a stick prep kit with chlorhexidine. The cranial access kit that comes with the monitoring device typically comes with a standard drape and additional sterile supplies to create a field of sterility. Alternatively, sterile towels, adherent plastic dressings, and other basic drapes may be used.

6.6.4 Incision and Twist Drill

Local anesthetic such as lidocaine with epinephrine is injected at the incision site. A stab incision is made with a #15 blade. The hand crank drill is then used to make a hole perpendicular to the skull surface. Once the inner table is

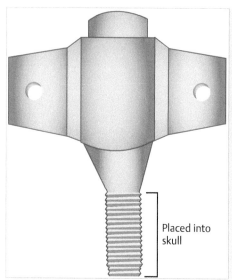

Fig. 6.3 Monitor anchor/bolt. The anchoring bolt secures the device into bone with metal threads which are hand screwed in place. The top of the anchor has an entry point for the probes. Anchors are typically multi-lumen when used in PbtO$_2$ monitoring systems, thus allowing for multiple parameters to be checked through the same anchor.

Placed into skull

opened, the drill is withdrawn. The bony debris is irrigated away with a syringe of water. A guiding anchor (bolt) is threaded into the entry site and manually twisted until finger-tight (see ▶ Fig. 6.3).

6.6.5 Dural Opening

Prior to opening the dura, blood pressure should be evaluated and lowered, if necessary, to minimize the risk of intracranial hemorrhage. A spinal needle is then passed through the anchor and used to perforate the dura.

6.6.6 Probe Placement and Securement

Some devices must be calibrated to a "zero" point prior to insertion. This is typically accomplished by connecting the device to the console prior to insertion. The system is then calibrated to a "zero" point using the guidelines specific for a given system. For some devices, an obturator is used to create a pathway into the brain parenchyma. Next, the probe is inserted into the anchor and subsequently secured. Devices vary in terms of markings indicating depth of insertion. Typically, entry in the 2 to 4 cm range into the brain parenchyma is sufficient. In devices used for PbtO$_2$ monitoring, more than one probe will likely be used. The anchor/bolt may have multiple ports. Each of the probes is usually placed in its own lumen. The Licoxsystem has an ICP probe and a PbtO$_2$/temperature probe (see ▶ Fig. 6.4).

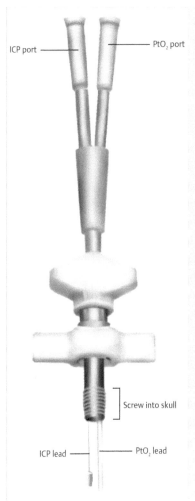

ICP port

PtO₂ port

Fig. 6.4 Licox monitor with probe ports. Shown are the two major components, consisting of an intracranial pressure (ICP) monitoring probe and a PtO₂/temperature probe.

Screw into skull

ICP lead   PtO₂ lead

6.6.7 Connection to Monitoring System

Following insertion, the device is connected to the console and initial metrics may be captured. It is necessary to allow approximately 1 hour for oxygen to diffuse into the cannula to obtain accurate measurements. If the operator feels there is a discrepancy between what is expected and measured, there should be an evaluation of the system to check for errors.

6.6.8 Closure and Dressing

A U-stitch suture may be placed at the scalp entry site to prevent cerebrospinal fluid (CSF) leakage around the anchor. Betadine-soaked gauze and/or plastic adhesive film dressings may also be applied.

6.6.9 Postprocedure Imaging

Postprocedure imaging typically includes a noncontrast CT of the head to ensure there is proper placement and no significant hemorrhage.

6.7 Complications

While there is a dearth of safety data for intraparenchymal oxygenation monitors, the reported rates of complications are quite low. In a review of safety data regarding the Licox device encompassing 292 patients, only 2 iatrogenic hematomas (neither of which required evacuation) and no infections were reported.[15] However, given the similarities between the hardware and insertion techniques of intraparenchymal oxygenation monitors and intraparenchymal ICP monitors, the more widely reported complications of the ICP monitors can guide further discussion. Specific complications and methods of avoidance are mentioned below, including hemorrhage, CSF leak at the site of device insertion, skull fracture secondary to burr hole drilling, and infection.

6.7.1 Hemorrhage

Case series have found the rate of hemorrhage associated with cerebral oxygenation monitoring is 0 to 2.0%, although these studies are small in size. A study of 1,000 patients with intraparenchymal ICP monitors found a rate of 2%. In patients with at least one abnormal coagulation parameter, the rate of hemorrhage was as high as 8%, which represents a significant risk factor.[16] Using correct insertion techniques, appropriate anatomic landmarks, and planning the insertion trajectory using CT scans to avoid major vessels and sinuses can reduce risk of hemorrhage.

6.7.2 CSF Leak

Leaking of CSF may occur around the monitor entry site. A simple nonabsorbable suture can help combat this. The suture is placed in a purse-string fashion and allows for a tighter interface between the scalp and the anchor device.

6.7.3 Skull Fracture

Although skull fracture is uncommon as a complication of monitor placement, it may occur secondary to drilling in the area of unstable calvarial bone (secondary to trauma). Careful assessment of the pre-procedure CT head with bone windowing should be performed to ensure the intended entry site does not come near a skull fracture. If a fracture occurs secondary to drilling, the clinician should be cautious of possible monitoring device displacement and/or epidural hemorrhage.

6.7.4 Infection

Infections have not been reported with cerebral oxygenation monitors, but it would be naïve to assume such infections do not occur. The risk of infection is likely similar to intraparenchymal ICP monitors and with similar risk factors. Reported infection rates of intraparenchymal ICP monitors are 0 to 0.8% and are associated with increased age, medical comorbidities, and systemic infection.[17] Infection risk can be reduced by using meticulous sterile technique, a single pre-procedure dose of appropriate antibiotics, and by removing the device as soon as possible.

6.8 Expert Suggestions/Troubleshooting

6.8.1 Sedation Issues

Common issues that may be encountered with sedation include patient movement and hemodynamic instability. When patients are intubated, deeper sedation is relatively easy and should be utilized to facilitate proper device placement. In nonintubated patients, the operator should keep an additional assistant present in case the patient begins to move. The secondary assistant may hold the patient while the primary assistant acquires more sedative medications. The operator should pause while patient comfort is re-established.

6.8.2 Positioning Issues and Tips

Head position and mobility is key. The head of the bed should allow ergonomic mobility of the operator's hands and easy access to the supply table. Some operators may place a small securing tape across the patient's forehead, out of the sterile field, to better "lock" the position. Rolled towels may also be placed on both sides to help immobilize the patient's head.

6.8.3 Scalp Bleeding and Avoidance

In the event of significant arterial bleeding from the scalp, it can be challenging to visualize the calvaria and for the operator to comfortably perform the procedure. A suture may be placed on the lateral side of the incision, parallel to it, and tied. This can tie off any bleeding vessels. Application of local anesthetic with a vasoconstrictive substance such as epinephrine is helpful. This should be applied at least 5 to 10 minutes prior to the incision (right before draping is optimal). This time-lag allows for the medications to decrease local blood flow.

6.8.4 Craniotomy Angulation and Tips

Remaining perpendicular to the scalp at all times, for each step of the procedure, is critical. Even small variations in angulation can lead to challenges in drilling and probe placement.

6.8.5 Dural Opening

It is preferable to open the dura with a spinal needle. This is typically performed in a careful manner to prevent the needle from penetrating deep into the brain. The operator should proceed slowly and ensure the dura is opened on the first insertion. Multiple insertions greatly increase the chances of hemorrhage.

6.8.6 Probe Pull-Out and Avoidance

Securing the probe with plastic adherent film dressings may be of utility, especially at potential "pull-out" points. Furthermore, securing the wiring directly to the patient (at the shoulder typically) with tape may also help. This simple step can help prevent lead pull-out especially in case of patient agitation.

6.9 Conclusion

Brain tissue oxygenation (PbtO$_2$) monitoring is a useful tool in the management of neurocritical care patients. It provides a more direct assessment of the metabolic status of local tissue than measuring ICP and CPP alone. Intraparenchymal PbtO$_2$ sensors are inserted similar to intraparenchymal ICP monitors and are equally safe. Complications from device insertion are rare and can be further reduced with proper insertion technique.

References

[1] Bergsneider M, Hovda DA, Shalmon E, et al. Cerebral hyperglycolysis following severe traumatic brain injury in humans: a positron emission tomography study. J Neurosurg. 1997; 86(2): 241–251

[2] Eriksson EA, Barletta JF, Figueroa BE, et al. The first 72 hours of brain tissue oxygenation predicts patient survival with traumatic brain injury. J Trauma Acute Care Surg. 2012; 72(5):1345–1349

[3] Chang JJ, Youn TS, Benson D, et al. Physiologic and functional outcome correlates of brain tissue hypoxia in traumatic brain injury. Crit Care Med. 2009; 37(1):283–290

[4] Stiefel MF, Udoetuk JD, Spiotta AM, et al. Conventional neurocritical care and cerebral oxygenation after traumatic brain injury. J Neurosurg. 2006; 105(4):568–575

[5] Bardt TF, Unterberg AW, Härtl R, Kiening KL, Schneider GH, Lanksch WR. Monitoring of brain tissue PO_2 in traumatic brain injury: effect of cerebral hypoxia on outcome. Acta Neurochir Suppl (Wien). 1998; 71:153–156

[6] Valadka AB, Gopinath SP, Contant CF, Uzura M, Robertson CS. Relationship of brain tissue PO_2 to outcome after severe head injury. Crit Care Med. 1998; 26(9):1576–1581

[7] van den Brink WA, van Santbrink H, Steyerberg EW, et al. Brain oxygen tension in severe head injury. Neurosurgery. 2000; 46(4):868–876, discussion 876–878–. PMID: 10764260

[8] Narotam PK, Morrison JF, Nathoo N. Brain tissue oxygen monitoring in traumatic brain injury and major trauma: outcome analysis of a brain tissue oxygen-directed therapy. J Neurosurg. 2009; 111(4):672–682

[9] Spiotta AM, Stiefel MF, Gracias VH, et al. Brain tissue oxygen-directed management and outcome in patients with severe traumatic brain injury. J Neurosurg. 2010; 113(3):571–580

[10] Martini RP, Deem S, Yanez ND, et al. Management guided by brain tissue oxygen monitoring and outcome following severe traumatic brain injury. J Neurosurg. 2009; 111(4):644–649

[11] Green JA, Pellegrini DC, Vanderkolk WE, Figueroa BE, Eriksson EA. Goal directed brain tissue oxygen monitoring versus conventional management in traumatic brain injury: an analysis of in hospital recovery. Neurocrit Care. 2013; 18(1):20–25

[12] McCarthy MC, Moncrief H, Sands JM, et al. Neurologic outcomes with cerebral oxygen monitoring in traumatic brain injury. Surgery. 2009; 146(4):585–590, discussion 590–591

[13] Huschak G, Hoell T, Hohaus C, Kern C, Minkus Y, Meisel HJ. Clinical evaluation of a new multiparameter neuromonitoring device: measurement of brain tissue oxygen, brain temperature, and intracranial pressure. J Neurosurg Anesthesiol. 2009; 21(2):155–160

[14] Kett-White R, Hutchinson PJ, Al-Rawi PG, Gupta AK, Pickard JD, Kirkpatrick PJ. Adverse cerebral events detected after subarachnoid hemorrhage using brain oxygen and microdialysis probes. Neurosurgery. 2002; 50(6):1213–1221, discussion 1221–1222

[15] Maloney-Wilensky E, Gracias V, Itkin A, et al. Brain tissue oxygen and outcome after severe traumatic brain injury: a systematic review. Crit Care Med. 2009; 37(6):2057–2063

[16] Gelabert-González M, Ginesta-Galan V, Sernamito-García R, Allut AG, Bandin-Diéguez J, Rumbo RM. The Camino intracranial pressure device in clinical practice: assessment in a 1000 cases. Acta Neurochir (Wien). 2006; 148(4):435–441

[17] Tavakoli S, Peitz G, Ares W, Hafeez S, Grandhi R. Complications of invasive intracranial pressure monitoring devices in neurocritical care. Neurosurg Focus. 2017; 43(5):E6

7 Jugular Bulb Oxygen Monitor

Amanda Carpenter and Brent Lewis

Abstract

Early identification of dysfunctional oxygenation can prevent secondary brain injury. Jugular venous oximetry provides an indirect idea of oxygen use by the brain–it is used to determine the global balance of cerebral oxygen delivery and consumption. To obtain these measurements, a central venous catheter is inserted into the jugular bulb and a continuous jugular venous oxygen saturation (SjO_2) is recorded. The monitor is inserted via a seldinger technique to reach the jugular bulb. Ideal placement of the catheter is at the lower border of C1, and placement can be confirmed on x-ray.

Keywords: traumatic brain injury, jugular bulb, subarachnoid hemorrhage, neurocritical care, jugular venous oximetry

7.1 Introduction

Mitigation of secondary injury in the brain after a neurologic insult is one of the primary goals of neurocritical care. Dysfunctional oxygenation of brain tissue is an important cause of such secondary injury.

Cerebral oximetry encompasses a range of monitoring modalities to assess (directly or indirectly) the oxygenation status of the brain. These modalities include direct brain tissue oxygen ($PbtO_2$) monitoring (discussed in Chapter 6), microdialysis monitoring of extracellular glutamate and other molecules, near-infrared spectroscopy (NIRS) measurement of regional brain tissue oxygen saturation, and jugular bulb oxygen saturation (SjO_2) monitoring.

Here, we discuss the technique for insertion of an SjO_2 monitor. Of the aforementioned cerebral oximetry modalities, only SjO_2 monitoring is recommended by current professional guidelines.[1]

Jugular venous oximetry provides an indirect assessment of oxygen use by the brain—it is used to determine the global balance of cerebral oxygen delivery and consumption.

Jugular venous oximetry can be performed intermittently or continuously. Intermittent SjO_2 monitoring entails the insertion of retrograde jugular catheter with subsequent periodic aspiration and laboratory analysis of blood samples from the jugular bulb. Here, we describe the technique for continuous SjO_2 monitoring which is accomplished by insertion of a fiber-optic catheter with an SjO_2 monitor situated within the jugular bulb. For this latter technique, aspiration and laboratory analysis of blood is only required for calibration.

Jugular venous oximetry is a relatively noninvasive, cost-effective, and reliable tool in the armamentarium of critical care physicians.

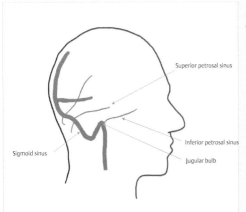

Fig. 7.1 Inferior skull base venous anatomy.

Superior petrosal sinus

Inferior petrosal sinus

Sigmoid sinus

Jugular bulb

7.2 Relevant Anatomy and Physiology

Blood from the brain drains mainly through the sigmoid and inferior petrosal sinuses into the internal jugular veins, as seen in ▶ Fig. 7.1. The jugular bulb is the connection between these sinuses and the internal jugular vein, and drains about 70% of the blood from the ipsilateral hemisphere, and 30% from the contralateral hemisphere. To monitor SjO_2, the tip of the fiber-optic catheter is placed into the jugular bulb, conventionally on the side with dominant drainage. Dominance can be determined radiographically by measuring the jugular foramina on computed tomography (CT) scan or functionally, if an intracranial pressure (ICP) monitor is present, by alternatingly compressing both jugular veins and observing the extent of increase in ICP. The right jugular venous pathway is dominant 80% of the time.

The arteriovenous oxygen content difference of the brain ($AVDO_2$) is calculated according to the following formula:

$$AVDO_2 = Hgb \times 1.34(SaO_2 - SjO_2) + 0.003(PaO_2 - PjO_2)^2$$

Cerebral oxygen extraction (CO_2E), a simplified representation of $AVDO_2$, is calculated according to the following formula:

$$CO_2E = SaO_2 - SjO_2$$

Saturation of arterial blood (SaO_2) is measured by continuous pulse oximetry, and saturation of jugular bulb blood (SjO_2) is measured continuously by the fiber-optic jugular bulb catheter.

Any disturbance that increases cerebral oxygen consumption or decreases oxygen delivery may decrease SjO_2. Current guidelines define SjO_2 < 50% as pathologic and harmful.[1] $SjO_2 > 75\%$ is also correlated with adverse outcomes in head injury.[3] Thus, the brain tissue of a healthy person extracts between 25 and 50% of arterial oxyhemoglobin, yielding a normal SjO_2 of 50 to 75%.

One prospective study showed mortality benefit by maintaining CO_2E between 24 and 42%.

High CO_2E suggests low cerebral blood flow relative to metabolic demand. This could be caused by decreased oxygen supply due to anemia, hypotension, or hypoxemia, or due to increased demand due to agitation, fever, seizures, or pain. This state has been described as "oligemic cerebral hypoxia," and can lead to ischemia.

Low CO_2E suggests that there is excess blood flow relative to metabolic demand, due to excessive cardiac output, or due to processes such as infarction, deep coma, or hypothermia causing decreased metabolism. This state of "luxury perfusion," can cause intracranial hypertension or hemorrhage.

Limitations of SjO_2 monitoring include erroneous values due to the monitor coming into contact with the vessel wall, thrombosis on the catheter tip, and the fact that it is a global monitor and may not detect regional ischemia or hyperemia.

7.3 Indications

In patients with traumatic brain injury and other critical neurosurgical illness (i.e., those with subarachnoid hemorrhage), measurement of SjO_2 can provide important information about the balance between cerebral oxygen supply and demand, and is used to guide physiologically based management.[1] There are also reports of using SjO_2 monitoring for patients undergoing cardiopulmonary bypass to optimize brain perfusion and limit the risk of post-bypass cognitive dysfunction.[4]

7.4 Contraindications

- Coagulopathy, thrombocytopenia, recent antiplatelet therapy, uremic platelet dysfunction, and recent thrombolytic therapy are relative contraindications.
- Insertion can be difficult in patients with neck trauma, cervical spine injuries, or tracheostomy.
- Local soft tissue infection in the neck or untreated bacteremia precludes insertion.

7.5 Equipment

- 4.0 French catheter with a fiber-optic oxygen saturation monitor
- 5.0 French introducer catheter tray which generally includes: 5.0 French introducer sheath, marked guidewire, dilator, access needle, syringes,

lidocaine, ChloraPrep, silk suture, serrated hemostat, 22- and 25-gauge needles, scalpel, gauze, drapes, saline-filled syringes, gown, hair net, and mask
- Postprocedure X-ray for placement verification

7.6 Technique

- Dominant internal jugular vein should be identified and procedure planned for that side.
- Patient should be positioned in Trendelenburg position with head turned to the opposite side (if there is no cervical spine injury).
- Anesthesia such as versed or fentanyl can be administered, if necessary.
- Site is prepped with sterile solution (i.e., 2% chlorhexidine gluconate).
- Operator gowns and then drapes the neck in sterile fashion.
- Lidocaine can be used as local anesthesia.
- Ultrasound guidance is used to find the internal jugular vein in between the sternal and clavicular heads of the sternocleidomastoid muscle.
- Puncture aspiration is performed with an 18-gauge needle on a syringe in a cephalic direction.
- Once in the vessel, Seldinger technique is used to pass a guidewire through the needle in a cephalic direction. It is important that the tip of the guidewire is J-shaped and is advanced only 6 to 8 cm beyond the site of needle insertion.
- The needle is then removed.
- The dilator and introducer sheath are advanced together over the wire into the vessel with a twisting motion.
- The dilator is then removed.
- The catheter is then inserted through the introducer until resistance is met (typically 17–18 cm), and then withdrawn 0.5 to 1 cm to avoid injury to the jugular bulb and to reduce risk of occlusion of the catheter tip.
- Ideal placement of the catheter is at the lower border of C1, and placement can be confirmed on lateral X-ray.
- The catheter should be sutured into place.

7.7 Complications

- Carotid artery puncture
- Jugular vein thrombosis
- Hematoma
- Line infection

7.8 Expert Suggestions/Troubleshooting

- To calibrate a fiber-optic SjO_2 monitor, blood must be aspirated from the jugular bulb for laboratory analysis. If the rate of aspiration is > 2 mL/min, then there can be considerable contamination from the extracranial vessels, yielding artificially high SjO_2 values.[5]
- SjO_2 monitoring is of limited value in patients with infratentorial pathology, as the majority of blood in the jugular bulb comes from the supratentorial compartment.

References

[1] Carney N, Totten AM, O'Reilly C, et al. Guidelines for the Management of Severe Traumatic Brain Injury. 4th ed. Brain Trauma Foundation; 2016

[2] Le Roux PD, Newell DW, Lam AM, Grady MS, Winn HR. Cerebral arteriovenous oxygen difference: a predictor of cerebral infarction and outcome in patients with severe head injury. J Neurosurg. 1997; 87(1):1–8

[3] Cormio M, Valadka AB, Robertson CS. Elevated jugular venous oxygen saturation after severe head injury. J Neurosurg. 1999; 90(1):9–15

[4] Schell RM, Kern FH, Greeley WJ, et al. Cerebral blood flow and metabolism during cardiopulmonary bypass. Anesth Analg. 1993; 76(4):849–865

[5] Matta BF, Lam AM. The rate of blood withdrawal affects the accuracy of jugular venous bulb: oxygen saturation measurements. Anesthesiology. 1997; 86(4):806–808

8 Central Line

Ahmed M. Meleis and John W. Liang

Abstract

Centrally inserted central venous catheters, or "central lines," are a common and useful tool in the Neuro-ICU. Here the following topics related to insertion of central lines are discussed in detail: relevant anatomy and physiology, indications/contraindications, equipment, technique, complications, and expert suggestions.

Keywords: access, central venous catheter, intravenous, jugular, femoral, subclavian

8.1 Introduction

Securing central venous access is a fundamental skill essential to the care of critically ill patients. In the United States, over 5 million central venous access catheters are placed annually[1] and on average remain in place for 7 to 10 days. Centrally inserted central venous catheters (CICVCs), or "central lines" as they are commonly known, may be placed in the subclavian, internal jugular, or femoral vein.[2][3] The concept of central line placement was first introduced by Dr. Werner Forssmann when he self-inserted a ureteric catheter through his cubital vein into his right heart.[7]

8.2 Anatomy/Physiology

Central venous access catheters are placed into a large vein in the body, terminating in the veins within the thorax. The three most common types of central lines placed are subclavian, internal jugular, and femoral. The catheter tip of a central line terminates in the superior vena cava for subclavian and internal jugular vein (IJV) central lines, and inferior vena cava for femoral central lines.

8.2.1 Subclavian Vein Anatomy

The subclavian vein is an extension of the axillary vein that originates at the outer border of the first rib. The vein runs under the clavicle, where it connects to the IJV to form the innominate, or brachiocephalic vein. The subclavian vein measures between 1 to 2 cm in diameter; however, it can be smaller or larger depending on the individual. The subclavian vein follows the subclavian artery and is separated from the subclavian artery by the insertion of the anterior scalene. Thus, the subclavian vein lies anterior to the anterior scalene while the subclavian artery lies posterior to the anterior scalene and anterior to the middle scalene.[11] The anatomy of the subclavian vein and surrounding structures is depicted in ▶ Fig. 8.1.

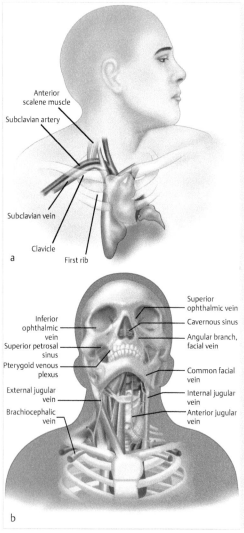

Fig. 8.1 (a, b) Anatomy of subclavian vein and surrounding structures.

8.2.2 Internal Jugular Vein Anatomy

The IJV is formed by the confluence of the inferior petrosal sinus and the sigmoid sinus. The IJV descends in the carotid sheath with the internal carotid artery. The vagus nerve (CN X) lies between the two. After receiving tributaries from the face and neck, the IJV continues to descend into the thorax, usually between the heads of the sternocleidomastoid muscle, before uniting with the subclavian vein to form the brachiocephalic vein.[11] The anatomy of the jugular vein and surrounding structures is depicted in ▶ Fig. 8.2.

8.2.3 Femoral Vein Anatomy

The femoral vein is the main deep vein of the lower limb, and travels next to the superficial femoral artery and common femoral artery. The femoral vein forms the continuation of the popliteal vein at the adductor opening, and becomes the external iliac vein as it ascends posterior to the inguinal ligament. In the distal adductor canal, the vein is posterolateral to the superficial femoral artery. Proximally in the canal, the vein lies posterior to the artery in the distal femoral

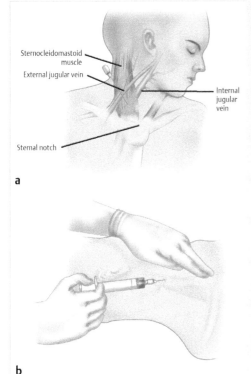

Fig. 8.2 (a, b) Anatomy of jugular vein and surrounding structures.

Sternocleidomastoid muscle

External jugular vein

Internal jugular vein

Sternal notch

a

b

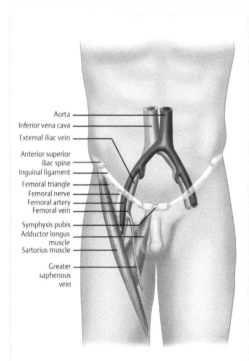

Fig. 8.3 Anatomy of femoral vein and surrounding structures.

Aorta
Inferior vena cava
External iliac vein
Anterior superior iliac spine
Inguinal ligament
Femoral triangle
Femoral nerve
Femoral artery
Femoral vein
Symphysis pubis
Adductor longus muscle
Sartorius muscle
Greater saphenous vein

triangle and medial to the artery at the base of the triangle. In the upper thigh, the vein is between the common femoral artery and femoral canal and therefore occupies the middle compartment of the femoral sheath.[12] The anatomy of the femoral vein and surrounding structures is depicted in ▶ Fig. 8.3.

8.3 Indications

There are a few generally agreed upon indications for placing a central line. These include:
• Inadequate peripheral venous access
• Rapid fluid resuscitation (requires an introducer sheath or other large bore catheter)
• Special drug administration such as vasopressors or hypertonic saline
• Need for total parenteral nutrition administration
• Invasive hemodynamic monitoring
• Pulmonary artery catheter placement
• Transvenous pacing
• Renal replacement therapy[8]
• Intravascular cooling

8.4 Contraindications

The following are relative contraindications to central line insertion:
• Coagulopathy, platelet dysfunction, and thrombocytopenia
• Local infection at site of placement (i.e., cellulitis)
• Thrombosis or stenosis of vein to be accessed
• Traumatized or burned site of insertion

The following are relative contraindications specific to subclavian central line insertion:
• Hemothorax or pneumothorax contralateral to the insertion site
• Tenuous pulmonary status

8.5 Equipment

To begin with, each intensive care unit (ICU) should have a central line "kit" that should be available at any time. Specific equipment will vary depending on the type of catheter being inserted. The following equipment is used for the insertion of a nontunneled triple lumen central line:

1. Sterile gown
2. Sterile gloves
3. Ultrasound probe cover/gel
4. 1% lidocaine with two syringes and needles (22 and 25 gauge)
5. 18-gauge introducer needle with 5 mL syringe
6. Guidewire
7. Triple-lumen indwelling catheter 7 French, 20 cm
8. Tissue dilator
9. Sterile flushes
10. End caps
11. Catheter clamp and fastener
12. Antibacterial patch
13. Scissors
14. Needle driver
15. Occlusive dressing
16. Gauze
17. 3.0 silk suture

8.5.1 Catheter Types

Central venous catheters may be tunneled or nontunneled. Tunneled catheters are used when it is anticipated that the catheter will be needed for longer than 3 to 4 weeks. Tunneled catheters have a lower rate of infectious complications[9] because of the distance between the skin entry site and the venotomy. Although they provide reliable long-term access, their complications include thrombosis, occlusion, and infection.[10] Nontunneled catheters are primarily used for short-term access in the emergency department, operating room, and ICU. These types of catheters are generally easier to place than tunneled catheters.[9] Nontunneled catheters have a higher rate of infectious complications and should generally be removed or exchanged after 5 to 7 days.[11]

There are many different models of central venous catheters, including single, dual, and triple lumen catheters, as well as introducer sheaths. Triple lumen catheters are generally preferred for ICU patients requiring multiple ports of access for medication administration. Introducer sheaths are required for rapid fluid resuscitation, transvenous pacing, or insertion of a pulmonary artery catheter. Specialized catheters with at least two large diameter ports are required for renal replacement therapy.

8.6 Technique

The steps below pertain to the insertion of a nontunneled triple lumen central venous catheter.

General steps for ultrasound-guided placement:

1. Connect ultrasound machine to a power source.
2. Select a linear vascular probe and confirm orientation (i.e., tap the left side of the probe and this should correspond with left side of the screen).
3. Examine target vein. Make sure vein is compressible, easily visualized, and centered on the screen.
4. Start with the short-axis view (probe perpendicular to the path of the vessel), as depicted in ▶ Fig. 8.4. Introduce the needle at a 45-degree angle and advance toward the vessel under direct visualization while applying gentle negative pressure to the syringe, as depicted in ▶ Fig. 8.5.

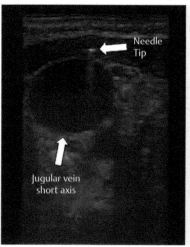

Fig. 8.4 Short-axis view of jugular vein and carotid artery.

5. Once the vessel is entered blood will fill the syringe. At this point the probe can be rotated 90 degrees so that it is parallel to the path of the vessel to obtain the longitudinal view, as depicted in ▶ Fig. 8.6. This view can help confirm the location of the needle and visualize the guidewire entry into the lumen of the vessel, as depicted in ▶ Fig. 8.7.

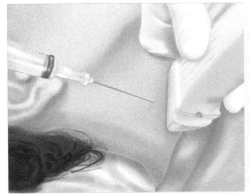

Fig. 8.5 Ultrasound guided puncture of jugular vein.

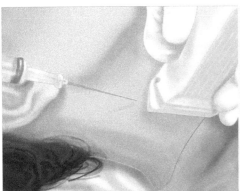

Fig. 8.6 Orientation of ultrasound probe for long-axis view.

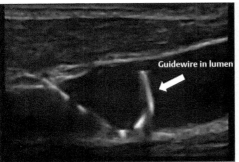

Guidewire in lumen

Fig. 8.7 Long-axis view of guidewire entering jugular vein.

8.6.1 Subclavian Vein Technique

Numerous landmarks have been described for determining the needle insertion site, as depicted in ▶ Fig. 8.8.[13,14,15] The following are some of the options mentioned, any of which will work:
- 1 cm inferior to the junctions of the middle and medial third of the clavicle
- Inferior to the clavicle at the deltopectoral groove
- Just lateral to the midclavicular line, with the needle perpendicular along the inferior lateral clavicle
- One finger breadth lateral to the angle of the clavicle

In general ultrasound guidance is not necessary for subclavian vein cannulation, although it may be helpful to inspect the vein with ultrasound prior to insertion to confirm that it is not stenotic or otherwise anatomically aberrant.
- Place the patient in Trendelenburg position and place a shoulder roll under the shoulder on the side of insertion. This will help elevate the chest area.
- Turn the patient's head to the contralateral side.

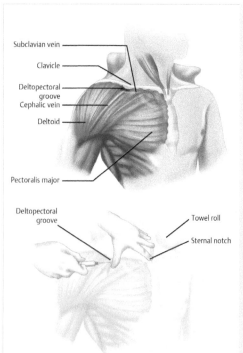

Fig. 8.8 Anatomic landmarks for cannulation of subclavian vein.

- Open the central line kit and confirm that all needed equipment is easy to reach for each step.
- Retract the curved J-tip wire into the plastic loop sheath to facilitate placement into the introducer needle.
- Flush the catheter and place caps on all lumens except the distal-most port which will need to remain open for passage of the guidewire.
- Sterilize the insertion site. The sterile area should be wide including the neck, chest, and shoulder.
- Don sterile mask, gown, and gloves.
- Drape the patient in a sterile fashion, with the insertion site exposed.
- Draw up the lidocaine 1% and infiltrate the skin, subcutaneous tissue, and the clavicular periosteum. It is especially important to anesthetize the periosteum as needle contact with the clavicle is the greatest source of pain during the procedure.
- Position the bevel of the introducer needle in line with the numbers on the syringe. While inserting the needle and syringe, orient the bevel upwards.
- Insert the introducer needle at the predetermined and chosen landmark; this is done while gently withdrawing the plunger of the syringe throughout the advancement.
- Once the needle makes contact with the clavicle, carefully depress the needle to slide it underneath the bone.
- Once under the clavicle, the needle should be carefully reoriented toward the suprasternal notch, aspirating on the syringe.
- A flash of venous blood indicates entry into the subclavian vein.
- When venous blood is freely aspirated, disconnect the syringe from the needle, and observe for steady, nonpulsatile flow of blood.
- If pulsatile arterial blood flow is observed, remove the needle and manually compress the infraclavicular fossa.
- If there is any uncertainty as to whether the vein or artery has been punctured, the needle can be connected to intravenous (IV) tubing in order to visually estimate or transduce the hydrostatic pressure in the vessel.
- After confirming puncture of the vein, insert the guidewire through the needle into the vein with the J-tip directed caudally.
- Advance the wire by approximately 30 cm (often indicated by three hash marks on many wires).
- The operator or an assistant should observe the patient's heart rhythm at this point in the procedure and the wire should be slightly withdrawn if there are premature ventricular contractions.
- Holding the wire in place, withdraw the introducer needle and place it in a safe location.
- One hand should remain on the wire at all times until it is withdrawn after placement of the catheter.

- Use a scalpel to make a small stab incision just against the wire to enlarge the catheter entry site.
- Thread the dilator over the wire and through the skin and subcutaneous tissue to a depth of several centimeters with a gentle twisting motion.
- Remove the dilator and thread the catheter over the wire until it exits the distal-most port.
- Grasp the wire and continue to thread the catheter to the desired depth. Generally, if entering the right subclavian vein, the length of catheter inserted should be 15 cm, and for the left subclavian vein it should be 18 cm.
- Once at target depth, remove the wire and place a cap on the distal-most port.
- Attach a syringe to each port and confirm that blood can be readily aspirated.
- Flush each port with saline.
- Suture the catheter in place and apply a sterile dressing.
- A chest X-ray should be obtained to confirm appropriate placement and to rule out pneumothorax.

8.6.2 Femoral Vein Technique

- Place the patient in the supine position, with the inguinal area exposed to allow proper identification of anatomic landmarks.[15,16,17]
- Open the central line kit and confirm that all needed equipment is easy to reach for each step.
- Retract the curved J-tip wire into the plastic loop sheath to facilitate placement into the introducer needle.
- Flush the catheter and place caps on all lumens except the distal-most port which will need to remain open for passage of the guidewire.
- Sterilize the insertion site.
- Don sterile mask, gown, and gloves.
- Drape the patient in sterile fashion, with the insertion site exposed.
- Identify the inguinal ligament and the femoral arterial pulsations. Identify a point approximately 1 cm below the inguinal ligament and 0.5 to 1 cm medial to the femoral arterial pulsation. This point is a safe access point for entry.
- Alternatively, ultrasound can be used to locate the vein.
- Gentle compression with the ultrasound transducer will differentiate the artery from the vein.
- Inject lidocaine 1% at the insertion site.
- If ultrasound guidance is not used, a small (26-gauge) exploratory or "finder" needle on a 5-mL syringe can be used to identify the vein and gain initial access.
- Enter the skin in an approximately 45 degrees cephalic direction, aspirating on the syringe throughout the process.

- As the vein is punctured, a flash of dark venous blood into the syringe indicates that the needle tip is within the femoral vein lumen.
- Place the larger needle immediately adjacent to the finder needle, and enter the femoral vein again and remove the finder needle.
- Thread the flexible J-tip guidewire through the lumen of the needle and into the vein lumen.
- Advance the guidewire until approximately one-third of its length is within the lumen of the vein.
- One hand should remain on the wire at all times until it is withdrawn after placement of the catheter.
- Make a small stab incision with a scalpel just against the wire to enlarge the catheter entry site.
- Thread the dilator over the wire and through the skin and subcutaneous tissue to a depth of several centimeters with a gentle twisting motion.
- Remove the dilator; then thread the catheter over the wire until it exits the distal-most port.
- Grasp the wire and continue to thread the catheter to the desired depth. For femoral vein insertion it is generally appropriate to insert the catheter to 20 cm or its maximum length.
- Once at target depth, remove the wire and place a cap on the distal-most port.
- Attach a syringe to each port and confirm that blood can be readily aspirated.
- Flush each port with saline.
- Suture the catheter in place and apply a sterile dressing.

8.6.3 Internal Jugular Vein Technique

- Place the patient supine in the Trendelenburg position with the head turned contralateral to the side of entry.
- Stand at the head of the patient's bed, facing the patient's feet.
- Sterilize the insertion site.
- The sterile area should be wide and include the neck, chest, and shoulder.
- Don sterile mask, gown, and gloves.
- Drape the patient in a sterile fashion, with the insertion site exposed.
- Apply acoustic gel on the linear transducer probe and identify the vascular structures in the neck (carotid artery and IJV). Apply slight pressure with the transducer in order to distinguish between the compressible IJV and the pulsatile carotid artery.
- Inject lidocaine 1% at the insertion site.
- Insert the introducer needle attached to an empty syringe at a 45 degrees angle to the skin, 2 cm cephalad to the position of the ultrasound probe while gently aspirating on the syringe.
- The needle should approximately be aimed at the ipsilateral nipple.

- Use the ultrasound probe to follow the tip of the needle toward the target vessel, redirecting as needed. It is easiest to follow the tip of the needle when the ultrasound probe is perpendicular to the needle. With the ultrasound, directly observe the needle tip as it enters the vessel.
- A flash of venous blood indicates entry into the IJV.
- When venous blood is freely aspirated, disconnect the syringe from the needle, and observe for steady, nonpulsatile flow of blood.
- If pulsatile arterial blood flow is observed, remove the needle and manually compress the carotid artery.
- If there is any uncertainty as to whether the vein or artery has been punctured, the needle can be connected to IV tubing in order to visually estimate or transduce the hydrostatic pressure in the vessel.
- After confirming puncture of the vein, insert the guidewire through the needle into the vein.
- Advance the wire by approximately 30 cm (often indicated by three hash marks on many wires).
- The operator or an assistant should observe the patient's heart rhythm at this point in the procedure and the wire should be slightly withdrawn if there are premature ventricular contractions.
- Holding the wire in place, withdraw the introducer needle and place it in a safe location.
- One hand should remain on the wire at all times until it is withdrawn after placement of the catheter.
- To further confirm that the wire is appropriately situated, the ultrasound can be used to visualize the wire within the vein in a long-axis view (parallel to the vessel).
- Use a scalpel to make a small stab incision just against the wire to enlarge the catheter entry site.
- Thread the dilator over the wire and through the skin and subcutaneous tissue to a depth of several centimeters with a gentle twisting motion.
- Remove the dilator and thread the catheter over the wire until it exits the distal-most port.
- Grasp the wire and continue to thread the catheter to the desired depth. Generally, if entering the right IJV, the length of catheter inserted should be 16 cm, and for the left IJV it should be 17 cm.
- Once at target depth, remove the wire and place a cap on the distal-most port.
- Attach a syringe to each port and confirm that blood can be readily aspirated.
- Flush each port with saline.
- Suture the catheter in place and apply a sterile dressing.
- A chest X-ray should be obtained to confirm appropriate placement and to rule out pneumothorax.

8.7 Complications

Complications of central line placement have been well-studied and described, including pneumothorax, hemothorax, and arterial injury. Infection remains a significant problem with central line placement despite sterile technique. Studies have reported infection rates ranging from 5 to 26% or from 2.9 to 11.3 cases per 1,000 catheter days.[4,5] Such infections may lead to bacteremia and sepsis. In addition to infection, venous thrombosis is a less-recognized complication of central line placement, with an incidence of 2 to 26%.[4] While not all such thromboses are symptomatic, they may complicate future venous access and may also result in late symptoms of venous claudication.[6]

In summary, some of the reported and known complications are:

- Pneumothorax
- Hemothorax
- Retroperitoneal hematoma
- Arterial injury
- Pseudoaneurysm
- Arteriovenous fistula
- Local hematoma
- Guidewire-induced arrhythmia
- Thoracic duct injury
- Guidewire embolism
- Air embolism
- Infection
- Vessel thrombosis
- Catheter fracture
- Vascular erosion

8.8 Expert Suggestions/Troubleshooting

- Arrange equipment in the order it will be used.
- Flush all catheter ports with saline at the beginning of the procedure.
- Do not place a cap over the distal-most port initially, as this will need to remain open for passage of the guidewire.
- Do not force the guidewire. If it is not threading through, it is best to reattach the syringe, remove needle, and try a different trajectory.
- Before moving to a different side (i.e., right subclavian after previously attempting left subclavian), obtain a chest X-ray to ensure that there is no pneumothorax on the previously attempted side.
- Administer appropriate analgesia and sedation as required on a case-by-case basis.
- Sometimes, visual inspection of how dark or bright the blood appears or the rate at which it flows out of the introducer needle may be misleading. It is

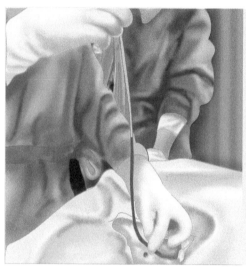

Fig. 8.9 Manual assessment of blood pressure to confirm venous placement.

advisable to confirm you are indeed in a vein prior to dilating the vessel. This can be done by attaching a sterile tubing to the needle and using it as a make-shift manometer, as depicted in ► Fig. 8.9.

- When inserting a subclavian central line in an intubated patient, note the baseline heart rate, respiratory rate, and peak airway pressure. Significant increase from baseline in these parameters may be due to pneumothorax.

References

[1] Mermel LA, Farr BM, Sherertz RJ, et al. Infectious Diseases Society of America, American College of Critical Care Medicine, Society for Healthcare Epidemiology of America. Guidelines for the management of intravascular catheter-related infections. J Intraven Nurs. 2001; 24(3):180–205

[2] Parienti JJ, Thirion M, Mégarbane B, et al. Members of the Cathedia Study Group. Femoral vs jugular venous catheterization and risk of nosocomial events in adults requiring acute renal replacement therapy: a randomized controlled trial. JAMA. 2008; 299(20):2413–2422

[3] Turcotte S, Dubé S, Beauchamp G. Peripherally inserted central venous catheters are not superior to central venous catheters in the acute care of surgical patients on the ward. World J Surg. 2006; 30(8):1605–1619

[4] McGee DC, Gould MK. Preventing complications of central venous catheterization. N Engl J Med. 2003; 348(12):1123–1133

[5] O'Grady NP, Alexander M, Dellinger EP, et al. Centers for Disease Control and Prevention. Guidelines for the prevention of intravascular catheter-related infections. MMWR Recomm Rep. 2002; 51 RR-10:1–29

[6] Ong B, Gibbs H, Catchpole I, Hetherington R, Harper J. Peripherally inserted central catheters and upper extremity deep vein thrombosis. Australas Radiol. 2006; 50(5):451–454

[7] Beheshti MV. A concise history of central venous access. Tech Vasc Interv Radiol. 2011; 14(4):184–185

[8] Bourgeois SL, Jr. Central venous access techniques. Atlas Oral Maxillofac Surg Clin North Am. 2015; 23(2):137–145

[9] Akaraborworn O. A review in emergency central venous catheterization. Chin J Traumatol. 2017;20(3):137-140.

[10] Cheung E, Baerlocher MO, Asch M, Myers A. Venous access: a practical review for 2009. Can Fam Physician. 2009; 55(5):494–496

[11] Whitaker RH, Borley NR. Instant Anatomy. Wiley-Blackwell; 2000 ISBN:0632054034

[12] Uflacker R. Atlas of Vascular Anatomy. Lippincott Williams and Wilkins; 2006 ISBN: 9780781760812

[13] Braner DA, Lai S, Eman S, Tegtmeyer K. Videos in clinical medicine: central venous catheterization—subclavian vein. N Engl J Med. 2007; 357(24):e26

[14] Kilbourne MJ, Bochicchio GV, Scalea T, Xiao Y. Avoiding common technical errors in subclavian central venous catheter placement. J Am Coll Surg. 2009; 208(1):104–109

[15] Brass P, Hellmich M, Kolodziej L, Schick G, Smith AF. Ultrasound guidance versus anatomical landmarks for subclavian or femoral vein catheterization. Cochrane Database Syst Rev. 2015; 1: CD011447

[16] Hoffman T, Du Plessis M, Prekupec MP, et al. Ultrasound-guided central venous catheterization: a review of the relevant anatomy, technique, complications, and anatomical variations. Clin Anat. 2017; 30(2):237–250

[17] Lee YH, Kim TK, Jung YS, et al. Comparison of needle insertion and guidewire placement techniques during internal jugular vein catheterization: the thin-wall introducer needle technique versus the cannula-over-needle technique. Crit Care Med. 2015; 43(10):2112–2116

9 Arterial Line

Irene Say, Celina Crisman, and Nitesh V. Patel

Abstract

Arterial lines cannulation is a common procedure in the intensive care unit (ICU). Here, the relevant anatomy, physiology, indications, technique, complications, and expert suggestions are outlined.

Keywords: arterial line, blood pressure, hypertension, hypotension, radial artery, mean arterial pressure, hemodynamic stability, intensive care unit

9.1 Introduction

Insertion of an arterial line entails the placement of a catheter in a patient's artery, most commonly the radial artery. An arterial catheter can be used to transduce continuous blood pressure measurements and to sample arterial blood for laboratory analysis. Accurate measurement of blood pressure is not only essential for managing cardiac output and monitoring ventilation in severe pulmonary disease, but also vital in guiding neurocritical care of diseases such as intracranial hypertension, intracranial hemorrhage, neurogenic shock, and cerebral vasospasm. Unlike noninvasive means of blood pressure management (NIBP), which is only episodic, the arterial line provides continuous, real-time measurement of blood pressure and gives convenient and immediate arterial access for blood sampling. Connection of the arterial catheter to an external transducer allows for quantitative measurement of intra-arterial blood pressure and an arterial waveform, representing the systolic and diastolic pulsations of the circulatory system. A typical arterial line schematic and radial artery anatomy are demonstrated in ▶ Fig. 9.1.

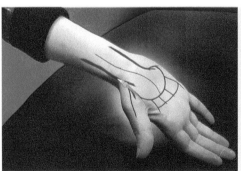

Fig. 9.1 A schematic of a typical radial artery line is illustrated here, with the underlying radial artery anatomy overlaid on the hand, showing associated collateral vasculature.

9.2 Anatomy/Physiology

The radial artery is most commonly accessed, followed by the femoral artery, predominantly because of its superficial anatomy and well-established low risk of complications.[1] Specifically, the radial artery is directly palpable on the skin, supplies the hand with collateral circulation, and, if compromised, does not typically lead to life-threatening complications. Other arteries, such as the femoral, dorsalis pedis, and brachial arteries may be cannulated, but present unique complications such as positional measurements, short life-span, or limb-threatening arterial thromboses. The axillary artery can usually be cannulated safely; however, ultrasound guidance is required.

9.3 Indications

Arterial lines are most frequently performed for continuous, real-time measurement of intra-arterial blood pressure and for providing reliable arterial access for frequent blood sampling.

9.3.1 Measurement of Intra-arterial Blood Pressure

Accurate measurement of blood pressure is vital in all neurocritical care patients. Continuous blood pressure measurement is a crucial component of the resuscitation of a patient in shock. Common scenarios of shock management in the Neuro-ICU would include hypovolemic shock due to severe blood loss, cardiogenic shock due to neurogenic stunned myocardium, neurogenic shock due to spinal cord injury, and septic shock. Conversely, monitoring and treatment of dangerously high blood pressure is equally important. In the Neuro-ICU, maintenance of normal blood pressure is vital to prevent further hemorrhage in a patient with a stroke, intracranial hemorrhage, or recent surgery.

9.3.2 Arterial Access for Frequent Blood Sampling

Frequent blood draws are often required in the ICU setting for both routine, daily laboratory studies, and for evaluating a patient's respiratory status through arterial blood gases (ABGs). However, in the Neuro-ICU, the arterial line is especially important for more frequent evaluation of laboratory parameters, such as the serum sodium (Na) (i.e., for patients with diabetes insipidus) or the serum osmolality (osm) (i.e., for patients with intracranial hypertension). Through an arterial line, one can avoid repeated puncture of an artery, which can lead to permanent damage, vasospasm, or even limb-threatening thrombosis.

9.4 Contraindications

Absolute contraindications for placement of an arterial line include impaired circulation to the hand, secondary to known traumatic, congenital, or rheumatologic etiology. Pre-procedural physical examination of both hands involves palpating a radial pulse, inspecting for previous surgical scars or overlying skin infection, and evaluating for adequate capillary refill. Coagulopathy and platelet dysfunction are relative contraindications:

- Previous radial artery damage or compromised circulation to the hand.
- No palpable pulse in the artery of interest.
- Severe coagulopathy, thrombocytopenia.
- Overlying skin infection.

9.5 Equipment

Prior to performing an arterial line, one must obtain skin antiseptic such as chlorhexidine, a cap and mask with eye shield, sterile gloves, sterile drapes, sterile gauze, sterile tegaderm, a securing nonabsorbable suture (nylon, silk) and needle introducer, guidewire, and catheter. We recommend using the Seldinger technique, in which an integrated catheter is threaded over the guidewire once the artery is cannulated. We have a Doppler ultrasound available, although not routinely used. Local fast-acting anesthetic, such as 1% lidocaine without epinephrine, is infiltrated at the proposed site of the arterial line in awake patients for comfort. Immediately prior to the procedure, the appropriate nursing staff is notified for arrangement of the pressure tubing and transducer once the arterial line is placed:

- Skin antiseptic (chlorhexidine, betadine)
- Cap, mask with eye shield, sterile gloves, and drapes/towels
- Arterial line kit (introducer needle, guidewire, 20G arterial line catheter)
- Nonabsorbable suture (3–0 nylon, silk) and associated needle-driver, forceps, and scissors
- Occlusive tegaderm
- Arterial line tubing
- 1% lidocaine without epinephrine (optional)

9.6 Technique

After evaluating the patient and obtaining the appropriate equipment, the Allen's test may be performed to evaluate for collateral circulation in the palmar branches of the hand, perfused by both the radial and ulnar arteries. The goal of this bedside test is to evaluate whether ulnar artery can fully perfuse the hand in the event of radial artery compromise. Digital pressure is first applied simultaneously on both the radial and ulnar arteries to mimic occlusion for about 3 seconds. If the patient is awake, he or she can squeeze his or her hand several times, making a fist, to drain blood from the hand to allow for better visualization of subsequent capillary refill. Then, pressure on the ulnar artery is released and the patient's fingers are examined for appropriate color and capillary perfusion. If perfusion does not return or timing to perfusion is over 3 seconds, the radial artery is considered to be insufficiently supplied by collateral circulation and an alternative site should be considered.

To access the radial artery, the patient's hand is positioned supine and gently dorsiflexed. Maintaining this position is critical for successful access. A small amount of tape well above and below the proposed site may be useful in an awake patient. The local anesthetic, introducer needle, guidewire, and catheter are opened from the arterial line kit onto the sterile field. The wrist, upper forearm, and palm are prepped and sterilely draped. Local anesthetic without epinephrine is infiltrated superficially above the puncture site for patient comfort. After wearing sterile gloves, palpate the radial artery just proximal to the wrist and use two fingers of your nondominant hand and isolate about a 1 cm space in between those two fingers as a puncture site. The introducer needle is held with the dominant hand and angled at approximately 30 degrees upwards from the wrist. The needle then gently punctures the skin in between the two fingers of the dominant hand, confirming the location of the pulsating artery. The needle is then advanced until a bright red flash is observed. At this point the angle of approach should be flattened and the needle is advanced an extra millimeter to situate it centrally within the lumen of the vessel. The guidewire is then threaded smoothly through the needle, well past the needle's length. The catheter is then threaded over the needle and guidewire with a gentle rotating motion via the Seldinger technique, and the needle and guidewire are removed. Pulsatile arterial flow will be immediately observed from the catheter and the arterial line catheter is then secured to the tubing and transducer. The catheter is secured with a nylon stitch at the catheter hub, along with occlusive tegaderm, and a small amount of gauze at the catheter hub. We do not typically utilize a dilator or stab incision for catheter placement, given the risk of damage to the radial artery. In agitated patients when reading is positional, we recommend securing the wrist in position with a stabilizing board underneath the wrist.

9.7 Complications

Placement of a radial artery arterial line is usually a safe, commonplace procedure in the operating room, interventional cardiology, neuro-interventional suites, and Neuro-ICU. The most common complication of a radial arterial line is a temporary arterial occlusion, which does not usually require treatment.[2] However, previous studies in the anesthesia, cardiac, and critical care literature have shown the following complication rates: 0.05% major bleeding and 1.4%

major vascular complications, including arterial thrombosis, potentially caus-ing ischemia to the hand.[3] Other less common risks include local and systemic infection, arteriovenous fistula formation, pseudoaneurysm, air embolism, and nerve injury.

9.8 Expert Suggestions/Troubleshooting

If no flash of arterial blood is observed after multiple attempts, consider using an ultrasound to locate the radial artery prior to attempting the procedure on the other hand. If a flash of blood is observed but no longer flows, the needle may either have become displaced out of (superficial to) the artery or could have punctured deep through the posterior wall of the artery. To troubleshoot this, begin by advancing the needle deeper. If pulsatile blood returns, drop the angle of approach and nudge the needle a hair deeper (< 1 mm) to position it centrally within the lumen of the vessel and then thread the guidewire. If no pulsatile blood is observed upon advancing the needle, gradually withdraw it. If there has been a through-and-through puncture, the needle tip will eventu-ally pass back through the lumen of the artery, at which point pulsatile blood will be observed and the guidewire can be threaded into the vessel.

Threading the catheter over the guidewire requires careful maneuvering and is best accomplished with a twisting motion. If multiple attempts to thread the catheter are unsuccessful, we recommend temporarily aborting the procedure to prevent vasospasm in the radial artery and holding pressure on the punc-ture site. We do not regularly dilate this access point to prevent damage to the artery. We assess the need for arterial lines daily and remove as soon as inva-sive blood pressure monitoring is no longer needed. Generally, we remove arterial lines after about 72 hours and consider an alternative site if further monitoring is needed.

If the radial artery is unable to be accessed, consider line placement in the axillary artery.

References

[1] Nuttall G, Burckhardt J, Hadley A, et al. Surgical and patient risk factors for severe arterial line complications in adults. Anesthesiology. 2016; 124(3):590–597

[2] Scheer B, Perel A, Pfeiffer UJ. Clinical review: complications and risk factors of peripheral arterial catheters used for haemodynamic monitoring in anaesthesia and intensive care medicine. Crit Care. 2002; 6(3):199–204

[3] Jolly SS, Amlani S, Hamon M, Yusuf S, Mehta SR. Radial versus femoral access for coronary angiography or intervention and the impact on major bleeding and ischemic events: a systematic review and meta-analysis of randomized trials. Am Heart J. 2009; 157(1):132–140

10 Cervical Traction

Michael Cohen, Irene Say, and Robert F. Heary

Abstract

Cervical traction is the placement of weighted cervical tongs commonly used to quickly reduce traumatic fracture-dislocations of the cervical spine and realign the cervical spine in awake and cooperative patients. Here, we first review the relevant anatomy and physiology, discuss indications and contraindications, and finally provide a step-by-step procedural guide with expert advice to avoid common pitfalls.

Keywords: cervical traction, spinal cord injury, closed reduction, spine trauma, halo vest, Gardner Wells tongs, cervical facet dislocation, Hangman's fracture, rotatory atlantoaxial subluxation

10.1 Introduction

Cervical traction is a technique used to restore proper cervical spine alignment and to achieve decompression of the cervical spinal cord by means of application of weight to the head. This is typically performed following a traumatic fracture or dislocation of the cervical spine. Tongs are applied to the head with metal screws that are inserted through the outer table of the skull. Weight is incrementally applied to the head to distract the cervical spine to restore cervical alignment.

Cervical traction is most commonly used as an initial adjunct treatment to restore cervical alignment prior to cervical fixation, either with internal stabilization and fusion or external fixation with a halo vest. Cervical traction can also be used intraoperatively to aid correction of alignment for degenerative cervical pathologies.

In this chapter, we describe the relevant anatomy and physiology of the cervical spine, discuss indications and contraindications for cervical traction, and review the appropriate equipment and technique of placing a patient in cervical traction.

10.2 Relevant Anatomy and Physiology

10.2.1 Cervical Spine Anatomy

The cervical spine has seven vertebral levels. C1 (atlas) and C2 (axis) have unique anatomic features that provide specialized functions. C1 is composed of a ring with lateral masses that give rise to superior facets that articulate with the occipital condyles and inferior facets that articulate with the C2 superior facets. C2 is composed of a large vertebral body, an odontoid process (dens), pedicles, a spinous process, laminae, transverse processes, and facets. A series of ligaments help stabilize the upper cervical spine and craniocervical junction during head and spine movement, including the atlanto-occipital, anterior longitudinal, transverse, apical, and alar ligaments.

The cervical spine segments below the C2 level are referred to as the subaxial cervical spine (C3–C7). Each segment in the subaxial cervical spine is composed of a vertebral body, pedicles, a spinous process, laminae, lateral masses, transverse processes, and facets. The subaxial cervical facet joints are oriented in the coronal plane (facing anterior) and angled approximately 45 degrees superiorly in the sagittal plane. The subaxial cervical ligaments can be organized into anterior and posterior groups. The anterior ligamentous complex includes the anterior longitudinal ligament (ALL) and the posterior longitudinal ligament (PLL). The posterior ligamentous complex (PLC) includes the ligamentum flavum, the interspinous ligaments, and the facet joint capsules.

10.2.2 Pathophysiology of Cervical Traction

The most common traumatic cervical injuries that would potentially require cervical traction are cervical facet dislocations, hangman's fractures, and displaced type II odontoid fractures. The common pathophysiology of all these fractures is the unstable malalignment of the normal cervical curvature with the potential to compress the cervical spinal cord. Cervical traction is intended to distract the cervical spine to reduce angulation, subluxation, or dislocation, which will align the fracture to promote bone healing and remove any compression on the spinal cord if present.

Cervical facet dislocations are typically caused by flexion injuries which "unlock" the facets, and in the process, allow them to dislocate. Cervical traction is applied such that the vector of force flexes and distracts the neck to again unlock the facet joints until they translate back to their anatomic position, at which point the vector of force can be neutralized. Hangman's fractures are typically caused by hyperextension injuries and cause forward angulation and distraction of C2 relative to the subaxial spine. Cervical traction is applied such that the vector of force is neutral or extend the neck slightly to reduce the angulation of C2. Similarly, anteriorly displaced or angulated type II odontoid fractures can be reduced using cervical traction with a vector of force providing gentle extension of the neck. Rotary atlantoaxial subluxation is a unilateral subluxation of the C1–C2 facet joint most often caused by severe muscle spasm in the neck. Pharmacological treatment of the muscle spasms and neutral cervical traction can usually restore normal anatomic alignment. Burst fractures of the subaxial cervical spine causing spinal cord compression can often be reduced with cervical traction provided the PLL is intact. Stretching the PLL with cervical traction can translate the fractured vertebral body ventrally away from the spinal cord.

10.3 Indications

Indications for cervical traction include: facet dislocations, displaced or angulated hangman's fractures, displaced or angulated odontoid fractures, rotary atlantoaxial subluxation, and subaxial burst fractures. Cervical traction is also used by some spine surgeons to provide distraction during anterior and posterior cervical fusions for degenerative cervical spondylosis and cervical spondylotic myelopathy. For the purposes of this chapter, we will focus only on traumatic indications for cervical traction.

10.3.1 Facet Dislocations

Cervical facet dislocation occurs when the inferior articular process (IAP) dislocates anterior to the superior articular process (SAP) of the subjacent level. If the IAP is directly above the SAP, the dislocation is called a "perched facet," whereas if the IAP is anterior to the SAP, the dislocation is called a "jumped facet." Facet dislocations can be unilateral or bilateral. Facet dislocation causes anterior subluxation of the superior vertebral body, leading to spinal canal stenosis and cervical cord compression. Spinal cord injury is common in cervical facet dislocation. In general, bilateral facet dislocations have a high incidence of complete spinal cord injuries, and unilateral facet subluxations tend to cause nerve root compression and radiculopathy. Flexion injuries such as motor vehicle collisions, falls from height, and diving accidents are common causes of cervical facet dislocations (▶ Fig. 10.1).

10.3.2 Displaced or Angulated Hangman's Fractures

Hangman's fractures, or traumatic C2 spondylolysis, are typically caused by hyperextension of the neck combined with an axial compression or distraction force. The fractured C2 pars interarticularis creates instability between C2 and C3 and anterolisthesis of C2 on C3 is frequent. Disruption of the PLL and C2–C3 disk can lead to anterior angulation of C2 (▶ Fig. 10.2). Treatment of angulated or displaced hangman's fractures is typically reduction followed by halo-vest immobilization for the more stable injuries and either an anterior C2–C3 anterior cervical discectomy and fusion (ACDF) or a posterior C1–C3 stabilization and fusion for the unstable injuries.

10.3.3 Displaced or Angulated Type II Odontoid Fractures

Type II odontoid fractures most commonly occur in elderly patients after simple falls from standing. However, they can also occur in younger patients after high-velocity hyperflexion or hyperextension injuries. Type II odontoid

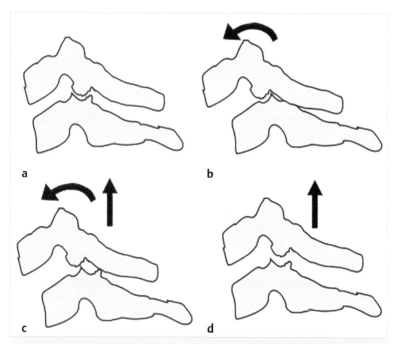

Fig. 10.1 Reduction of jumped facets. **(a)** Normal alignment of the facet joints. **(b)** A flexion-distraction injury causes facet dislocation, narrowing the spinal canal. **(c)** Cervical traction is used to distract the facet joints until they "unlock." **(d)** Normal alignment is restored.

fractures occur across the base of the odontoid process, where there is a vascular watershed zone due to the embryological growth of the blood supply to the dens. As a result of this poor blood supply to the base of the dens, there is a high rate of nonunion with nonoperative management. Type II odontoid fractures are commonly displaced or angulated anteriorly from hyperflexion injuries or displaced posteriorly from hyperextension injuries. These fractures are associated with transverse atlantal ligament injuries and are more likely to be unstable. Posteriorly displaced or angulated fractures can cause spinal cord compression and should be reduced urgently.

10.3.4 Rotary Atlantoaxial Subluxations

Atlantoaxial rotary subluxation (AARS) is a rotation of C1 on C2 associated with torticollis. This injury occurs most commonly in children. Although AARS can occur after significant trauma causing a fracture at C1 or C2, it is most common

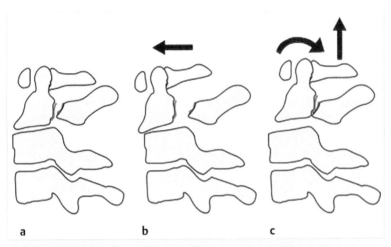

Fig. 10.2 Reduction of hangman's fracture. **(a)** A hangman's fracture. **(b)** Anterior subluxation of the fracture, causing narrowing of the spinal canal. **(c)** Cervical traction is used to distract and extend the cervical spine, translating the fracture back into alignment.

after minor injuries to the neck causing muscle strain, after surgery on the neck, or after infectious or inflammatory conditions involving the neck leading to prolonged muscle spasm. If no underlying fracture is found, AARS can be treated with analgesics, muscle relaxants, and collar immobilization if the subluxation is acute. Subacute and chronic AARS often require cervical traction and occasionally halo vest immobilization to successfully reduce.

10.3.5 Subaxial Burst Fractures

Burst fractures in the subaxial spine (C3–C7) involve loss of vertebral body height and retropulsion of the vertebral body into the spinal canal. This often causes spinal cord compression and injury. These fractures typically occur after high-energy axial compression injuries. Historically, cervical traction was used to decompress the spinal cord by applying tension on the PLL, thereby reducing the amount of bone retropulsion. Several studies have shown that cervical traction often produces incomplete decompression of the spinal cord.[1,2,3] The failure of traction to achieve reduction is usually the result of the PLL being disrupted. In cases where prompt reduction is not able to be successfully achieved, surgical decompression through an anterior cervical corpectomy or a posterior decompression and instrumented fusion have become more popular in the treatment of these injuries in patients with spinal cord injury.

10.4 Contraindications

Contraindications to cervical traction include clinically relevant skull fractures or diseases involving skull bone density such as Paget's disease of the skull or osteogenesis imperfecta, as skull pins may penetrate the skull. Young children under 3 years of age typically have skull sutures that have not yet fused and may be at increased risk during skull pin placement. As such, if traction is to be utilized in younger patients, consideration is given to utilizing a higher number of pins at a lower insertional torque through a halo ring. Atlanto-occipital dissociation (AOD) is a contraindication to cervical traction, as it is likely to widen the AOD and injure the upper cervical spinal cord and medulla. Traumatic brain injury that requires a craniotomy needs to be addressed before cervical traction is applied. Caution should be exercised when applying cervical traction in patients without a reliable neurological examination or with alterations in consciousness.

There is controversy regarding the presence of cervical disk herniation that could cause spinal cord compression while cervical traction is being applied. The incidence of disk herniation after traumatic cervical dislocation ranges from 8 to 42% in the literature.[4,5,6,7] While some centers rule out disk herniation with a pre-reduction magnetic resonance imaging (MRI) of the cervical spine, other centers routinely perform immediate closed reduction with cervical traction on awake patients with reliable neurological examinations prior to obtaining MRI. Those that advocate for immediate closed reduction cite the several-hour delay in spinal cord decompression associated with pre-reduction MRI, especially in patients with a potentially reversible spinal cord injury. Those that advocate for pre-reduction MRI cite the risk of iatrogenic disk protrusion during cervical traction that can lead to worsening neurologic deterioration.

Eismont et al published a series of 68 patients who underwent closed reduction with cervical traction with one neurological deterioration in their series.[4] Six patients were found to have disk herniations associated with their injuries and no awake patients in the series declined neurologically after closed reduction. Grant et al published a series of 82 patients who underwent early closed reduction with cervical traction prior to MRI. The incidence of disk herniation was 22% and one patient declined neurologically 6 hours after closed reduction.[5] Despite the presence of disk herniations, the authors found early closed reduction with cervical traction to be extremely safe when performed on awake patients who are cooperative with neurological examination. Rizzolo et al described 131 patients who underwent closed reduction with an 86% success rate and no neurologic worsening in any patient including those found to have disk herniations on MRI after reduction.[8] Vaccaro et al published a series of 11 patients, 2 with disk herniations prior to traction and 2 with new disk herniations after traction, with no neurologic deterioration in any patient after cervical traction.[9] At our institution, we have nearly immediate access to MRI and routinely attempt to obtain rapid-sequence T2 sagittal sequence to rule out disk herniation prior to closed reduction with cervical traction. However, we do not delay early closed reduction in awake patients with spinal cord injuries if there is a delay in obtaining MRI imaging.

10.5 Equipment

10.5.1 Gardner-Wells Tongs

Gardner-Wells tong is a C-shaped metal arch that fits around the head, typically made of stainless steel or graphite. The tongs have a hole on either end of the arch for skull pins to screw through. A metal ring is attached to the midpoint of the arch, where a rope can be tied to the tongs and run through a pulley system at the top of the hospital bed or stretcher that connects to weights which provide the traction (▶ Fig. 10.3).

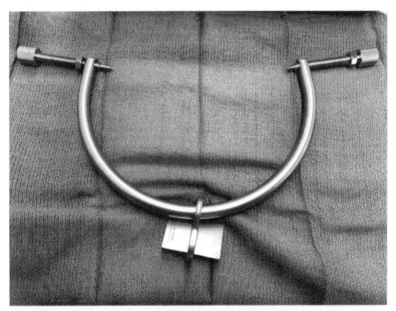

Fig. 10.3 Gardner-Wells tongs. For closed cervical traction, Gardner-Wells tongs are most commonly used to quickly reduce cervical facet dislocations. Bilateral pins are first prepped with bacitracin ointment, fixed at about 2 to 3 cm above the pinna, at the level of the external auditory canal, with slight posterior pin placement for flexion ligamentotaxis to realign the cervical spine. Pin sites are prepped with alcohol and infiltrated with local anesthetic, such as lidocaine. Pins are finger-tightened in opposing directions until the central metal pin indicator is flush with the pin. A posterior hook connects the tongs to the weights with a well-knotted rope at each end.

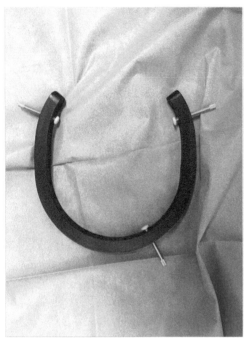

Fig. 10.4 Halo ring. The halo ring is typically connected to a halo vest for long-term cervical immobilization. Four sites, two anterior and two posterior, are secured with about 6 to 8 inch-lbs of torque. Anteriorly, pin sites are placed about 1 cm above the lateral eyebrow to avoid the supraorbital nerve and posterior pin sites are placed symmetrically opposite those pins. Pin sites are prepped with alcohol, infiltrated with local anesthetic, and all pins are prepped with bacitracin ointment. Pins are usually re-torqued 24 hours after initial placement, with either a torque wrench or break-off tabs, as per the specific halo brand manufacturer specifications.

10.5.2 Halo Ring

A halo ring fits circumferentially around the head and is typically fixed to the head using four skull pins (▶ Fig. 10.4). Typically, 6 to 8 foot-pounds of torque are utilized to secure the skull pins in an adult. The halo ring can be utilized instead of Gardner-Wells tongs and connected to a weight-pulley system to apply cervical traction. After closed reduction is accomplished using cervical traction, the halo ring can be connected to a halo vest to provide external fixation.

10.5.3 Modified Hospital Bed

A special hospital bed that counters the distracting force by bracing the shoulders is helpful to apply effective cervical traction. The Roto-rest bed is one example which includes shoulder braces to provide counter-traction and an integrated pulley system to hang weights (▶ Fig. 10.5).

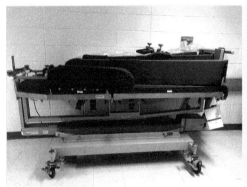

Fig. 10.5 Modified hospital bed. Patients in cervical traction must be placed in a modified hospital bed, which integrates the required weights and cervical traction device. Shoulder padding aids traction and visualization of the cervical spine during closed reduction.

10.5.4 Weight

Weights can be sequentially applied to the hooked weight-holder that is attached to the Gardner-Wells tong via a rope that turns 90 degrees as it bends around the pulley (▶ Fig. 10.6). Weights typically are in 2.5- and 5-lb increments. Multiple hooked weight-holders can be used if additional weight is required.

10.5.5 Halo Vest

The halo vest is an external fixation device that is fitted around the chest and rigidly secures the head and cervical spine in alignment (▶ Fig. 10.7). The halo vest can be used after closed reduction to maintain cervical alignment during transportation, advanced imaging such as MRI or myelogram, or until definitive internal fixation can be achieved. If excellent fracture alignment can be obtained using closed reduction, external fixation with a halo vest can be used to maintain alignment until definitive fusion occurs. Internal fixation has become increasingly popular as definitive treatment over the past several decades with advancements in spinal instrumentation, intraoperative monitoring, and neuro-navigation. External fixation with the halo vest remains an important option for patients at high risk for surgery. Definitive treatment with a halo vest is most often achieved in hangman's fractures or other injuries to the atlantoaxial complex. Lower cervical injuries often fail due to slippage of the alignment as a result of a phenomenon known as "snaking."[10]

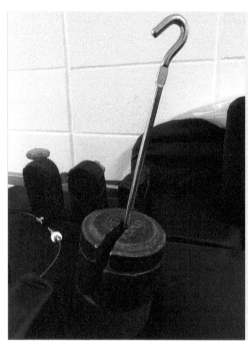

Fig. 10.6 Weight. Incremental weight, available in 2.5 and 5 lb metal discs, is hooked and stacked onto a metal weight-holder. This metal weight-holder is then hooked onto a rope, connected to the Gardner-Wells tongs.

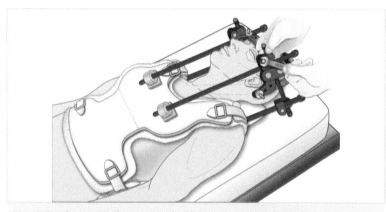

Fig. 10.7 Halo vest. The front and back of halo vest are applied separately and strapped together for a snug fit. The vest is connected to the halo ring through four longitudinal posts, which allow for additional custom cervical alignment. (Reproduced from Operative Procedure. In: Ullman J, Raksin PB, eds. Atlas of Emergency Neurosurgery. 1st Edition. Thieme; 2015.)

10.6 Technique

10.6.1 Patient Assessment

The initial assessment of a patient with cervical spinal trauma begins with evaluation of hemodynamic stability, especially given the possibility of neurogenic shock with cervical spinal cord injury. The patient should be placed in a rigid cervical collar. A focused history should be obtained to identify mechanism of injury, the possibility of other life-threatening injuries, and any pertinent medical or surgical history. A detailed neurological examination should be performed, including motor and sensory evaluation according to the American Spinal Injury Association (ASIA) classification.[11,12] If spinal cord injury is present, it should be classified as complete or incomplete as per the ASIA guidelines.

10.6.2 Tong Placement

The patient should be positioned supine and pin sites should be identified on either side of the skull, approximately 2 to 3 cm superior to the pinna of the ear. If neutral distraction is desired, the pin site is in-line with the external auditory meatus (EAM). However, if flexion or extension is desired, the pin site is adjusted slightly posterior or anterior to the EAM, respectively (▶ Fig. 10.8). The sites should be cleaned with alcohol and injected with local anesthetic.

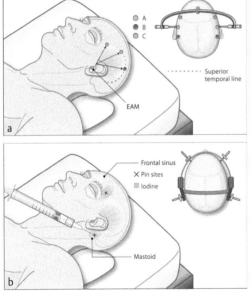

Fig. 10.8 (a, b) Placement of pins for Gardner-Wells tongs. Placement of pins at location "A" will result in neutral traction vector. Placement of pins at location "B" will distract in flexion (used for jumped facets). Placement of pins at location "C" will distract in extension (used for hangman's fractures). (Reproduced from Atlas of Emergency Neurosurgery. Ullman J, Raksin PB, eds. 1st Edition. Figure 11.3a. Thieme; 2015.)

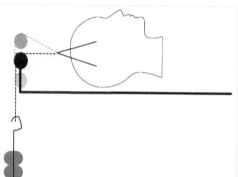

Fig. 10.9 Patient positioning and pulley adjustment. Illustration shows patient positioned on modified hospital bed with tongs applied to the head that are connected via a rope and pulley to a hooked weight-holder that hangs off the head of the bed. The pulley can be adjusted superiorly (*red*) to add a flexion force vector or inferiorly (*blue*) to add an extension force vector.

Low-dose narcotic or sedation can be given at this time, but the patient must be easily arousable and cooperative with a neurological examination at all times. The Gardner-Wells tongs are then placed in position and the skull pins are screwed into the skull simultaneously using both hands until the torque indicator protrudes above the plane of the surrounding cylinder.

10.6.3 Patient Positioning

Using strict cervical-spine precautions, the patient is placed supine and flat on a modified hospital bed equipped with shoulder braces and a weight-pulley system. The shoulder braces are fitted in place with extra padding if needed. The Gardner-Wells tongs are connected to the hooked weight-holder using a rope that runs through the pulley. The pulley height can be manipulated to alter the force vector of cervical traction. Raising the pulley will add flexion in addition to distraction, while lowering the pulley will add extension in addition to distraction (▶ Fig. 10.9).

10.6.4 Weight Application

A muscle relaxant can be judiciously administered to help relax the paraspinal cervical muscles; however, the patient must be awake and cooperative with frequent neurological testing. After a baseline neurologic examination and lateral portable X-ray of the cervical spine is obtained, initial weight (typically 5–10 lb) is applied to the hooked weight-holder.

Although many individuals anecdotally state that the maximum weight is 5 lb/level (i.e., 25 lb for a C5 burst fracture), there are also others who have utilized far greater weights to achieve reductions.[12] Weight is added in 5 lb increments every 10 minutes until reduction is achieved unless a radiographic or neurological change occurs that prohibits continued cervical traction.

Frequent fluoroscopic images assist in the safety of this procedure. A key step for high weight reductions is to immediately reduce the weight to 15 lb once a reduction has occurred.

10.6.5 Neurological Monitoring

Neurological examinations, checking motor and sensory functions, should be performed every 10 minutes prior to adding additional weight. Cervical traction should be discontinued if any decline in neurological function is detected and an MRI of the cervical spine immediately obtained. If the patient becomes lethargic or uncooperative with neurological examination, cervical traction should be discontinued. If cervical traction is discontinued prior to reduction, open reduction should be considered.

10.6.6 Radiographic Assessment

Portable lateral X-ray of the cervical spine is obtained at baseline and after each incremental weight addition (▶ Fig. 10.10). Alternatively, fluoroscopic images can be utilized for rapid imaging. Each X-ray is assessed for reduction of the fracture-dislocation as well as over-distraction of adjacent disk spaces. Cervical traction is discontinued and open reduction considered if over-distraction of adjacent disk spaces occurs prior to reduction. Computed tomography (CT) scanning can be utilized to assess reduction of the fracture-dislocation for cases in which X-ray is not clear. The patient may be placed in a halo vest after cervical traction is applied in order to obtain a CT scan. Further cervical traction can be performed after the CT scan is assessed by disconnecting the halo ring from the vest and re-applying weight.

10.7 Complications

Cervical traction is a safe and effective method to reduce certain fracture-dislocations of the cervical spine in awake and cooperative patients. The major risk of cervical traction is worsening a neurological injury that can occur from disk herniations, bone fragments, worsening alignment, or distraction injury of the spinal cord. These risks are greatly mitigated by incrementally adding small amounts of weight and frequently assessing for neurological or radiographic changes.

Cervical traction can frequently require large forces to be applied to the head to reduce fracture-dislocations. These forces, transmitted through the skull pins, can cause skull fractures and lacerations to the skin. The shoulder braces counter this force to allow for effective distraction, and the shoulders and paraspinal muscles are vulnerable to injury.

Fracture-dislocations of the cervical spine can cause injury or occlusion of the vertebral artery (VA). CT angiography can effectively diagnose VA dissection and occlusion, which is useful to know prior to applying cervical traction.

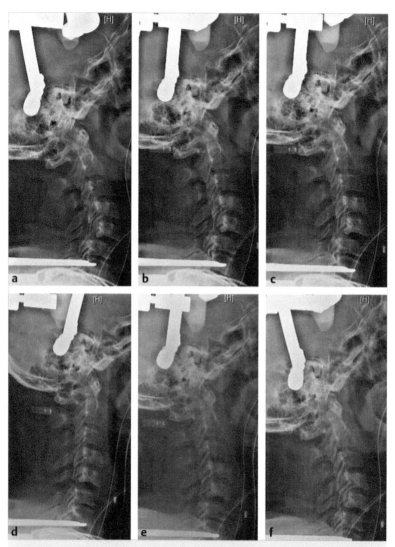

Fig. 10.10 Radiographic assessment of cervical traction. **(a)** Portable lateral X-ray showing C5–C6 facet dislocation prior to the application of cervical traction. **(b)** Minimal distraction of the C5–C6 disk space with 10 lb of weight. **(c)** Moderate distraction occurs at 20 lb of weight. **(d)** Significant C5–C6 disk distraction and "unlocking" occurs with 35 lb of weight. Gentle extension is added by adjusting the pulley and the weight is slowly diminished **(e)** until normal alignment is restored **(f)**.

Rapid reduction of the fracture-dislocation can lead to worsening VA dissection, embolism, and stroke.

10.8 Expert Suggestions/Troubleshooting

10.8.1 Resource Management

Cervical traction and halo application are a labor- and supply-intensive process. Extensive training is required to perform cervical traction and halo placement. There are many moving parts required for cervical traction and halo placement. It is most efficient to store all supplies together in a cart to prevent delays in reduction of a fracture-dislocation.

10.8.2 Halo Vest

The halo vest can be difficult to place on a patient with spinal cord injury and an unstable spine, especially once the patient is in cervical traction. If anticipating external fixation with a halo vest after cervical traction, we find it easiest to first log-roll the patient to place the back of the halo vest behind the patient, ensuring that the shoulder straps are high enough to reach around the front of the shoulders. After cervical traction is performed and reduction obtained, the front of the halo vest can be fixed both to the back of the vest and to the halo ring around the head. Once the halo system is fixed, cervical traction can be discontinued.

10.8.3 Force Vector

The direction of force applied during cervical traction is critical in effective reduction of fracture-dislocations of the cervical spine. The mechanism of injury and radiographic imaging must be carefully assessed to determine the appropriate force vector to be applied during cervical traction. Especially in jumped or perched facets, applying mild flexion along with distraction force during traction is necessary to unlock the facet joints in order to reduce the dislocation. Angulated odontoid or hangman's fractures may require an extension-distraction vector to re-align the fracture.

10.8.4 Converting to Open Reduction and Internal Fixation

As open reduction and internal fixation techniques have improved over the past several decades (spinal instrumentation, navigation systems, neuromonitoring), surgical fixation has become increasingly popular compared to external halo fixation. Typically, closed reduction with cervical traction is used as an emergent technique to reduce the fracture-dislocation and decompress the spinal cord prior to surgical fixation in the operating room. If excellent reduction and decompression are accomplished with closed reduction, often surgical fusion can be performed the following day in a more controlled manner. As most patients requiring cervical traction will end up going to the operating room either way, we have a low threshold for abandoning cervical traction and performing an emergent open reduction and internal fixation.

10.9 Conclusion

Cervical traction is a useful adjunctive treatment that can restore alignment of the cervical spine after traumatic fracture-dislocations. The primary treatment objective in spinal cord injury patients is rapid decompression of the spinal cord. Cervical traction can rapidly decompress the spinal cord and simultaneously simplify the surgical intervention to be performed.

References

[1] Koivikko MP, Myllynen P, Karjalainen M, Vornanen M, Santavirta S. Conservative and operative treatment in cervical burst fractures Arch Orthop Trauma Surg. 2000; 120(7-8):448–451

[2] Fisher CG, Dvorak MFS, Leith J, Wing PC. Comparison of outcomes for unstable lower cervical flexion teardrop fractures managed with halo thoracic vest versus anterior corpectomy and plating Spine. 2002; 27(2):160–166

[3] Kwon BK, Vaccaro AR, Grauer JN, Fisher CG, Dvorak MF. Subaxial cervical spine trauma J Am Acad Orthop Surg. 2006; 14(2):78–89

[4] Eismont FJ, Arena MJ, Green BA. Extrusion of an intervertebral disc associated with traumatic subluxation or dislocation of cervical facets. Case report J Bone Joint Surg Am. 1991; 73(10): 1555–1560

[5] Grant GA, Mirza SK, Chapman JR, et al. Risk of early closed reduction in cervical spine subluxation injuries J Neurosurg. 1999; 90(1, Suppl):13–18. Doi 10.3171/spi.1999.90.1.0013

[6] Sabiston CP, Wing PC, Schweigel JF, Van Peteghem PK, Yu W. Closed reduction of dislocations of the lower cervical spine J Trauma. 1988; 28(6):832–835

[7] Rizzolo SJ, Piazza MR, Cotler JM, Balderston RA, Schaefer D, Flanders A. Intervertebral disc injury complicating cervical spine trauma Spine. 1991; 16(6, Suppl):S187–S189

[8] Rizzolo SJ, Vaccaro AR, Cotler JM. Cervical spine trauma Spine. 1994; 19(20):2288–2298. Doi 10.1097/00007632-199410150-00007

[9] Vaccaro AR, Falatyn SP, Flanders AE, Balderston RA, Northrup BE, Cotler JM. Magnetic resonance evaluation of the intervertebral disc, spinal ligaments, and spinal cord before and after closed traction reduction of cervical spine dislocations Spine. 1999; 24(12):1210–1217

[10] Ivancic PC, Beauchman NN, Tweardy L. Effect of halo-vest components on stabilizing the injured cervical spine Spine. 2009; 34(2):167–175. Doi 10.1097/BRS.0b013e31818e32ba

[11] Maynard Jr FM, Bracken MB, Creasey G, et al. American Spinal Injury Association. International Standards for Neurological and Functional Classification of Spinal Cord Injury Spinal Cord. 1997; 35(5):266–274

[12] Cotler JM, Herbison GJ, Nasuti JF, Ditunno Jr JF, An H, Wolff BE. Closed reduction of traumatic cervical spine dislocation using traction weights up to 140 pounds Spine. 1993; 18(3):386–390

11 Intubation

John W. Liang, Elena Solli, and David A. Wyler

Abstract
Endotracheal intubation is a key skill in the neurointensivist toolbox. The neurocritical care patient demands additional attention to blood pressure and carbon dioxide control. It is important to be able to properly assess the patient's airway, have all essential equipment ready, and anticipate any potential difficulties during the procedure.

Keywords: airway, respiratory failure, intubation, endotracheal, oxygenation

11.1 Introduction

Securing and maintaining an airway is one of the most important components of resuscitation and critical care medicine. This chapter focuses on evaluation and management of the airway. While endotracheal intubation is typically the end goal, one must keep in mind that the skill of manually ventilating a patient is more important and often more difficult. Inability to ventilate a patient will bring panic to even the most seasoned practitioner. Therefore, all trainees should practice and develop good ventilation techniques (i.e., obtaining good seal with bag-valve mask) taught in Advanced Cardiac Life Saving courses before attempting intubation.

11.2 Relevant Anatomy/Physiology

Endotracheal intubation can be achieved orally or nasally. The oral route is more common and preferred. The nasopharynx joins the oropharynx near the base of the tongue. The vallecula is a cavity formed by the base of the tongue and the epiglottis and is used as a landmark for placing intubation blades/scopes. Best practice is to avoid lifting force while visualizing these landmarks as lacerations to the soft tissues may otherwise occur. The epiglottis is a cartilaginous flap attached to the larynx entrance and serves as a protective mechanism covering the larynx during swallowing to prevent food from entering the trachea and lungs (▶ Fig. 11.1). The larynx ends and the trachea begins at the level of the cricoid cartilage. The trachea continues down into the carina and bifurcates in the left and right main stem bronchi. The left bronchus is more angulated due to space taken up by the heart whereas the right bronchus is shorter and more vertical; thus the endotracheal tube, if advanced too far, is more likely to be in the right bronchus. Most providers perform intubations by positioning themselves at the head of the bed and often obtain a view as seen in ▶ Fig. 11.2.

Intubation

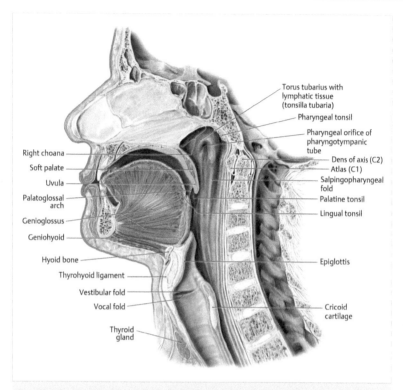

Fig. 11.1 Oral cavity. Artist's drawing of a midsagittal section of the oral cavity and pharynx. (Reproduced with permission from Schuenke et al., Atlas of Anatomy, © Thieme 2012, Illustration by Karl Wesker.)

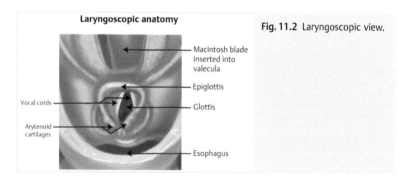

Fig. 11.2 Laryngoscopic view.

11.3 Indications

The primary indications for intubation can be broken down broadly into three categories: airway, lung, and tissue.

11.3.1 Airway

Airway management is the first priority in the time-honored "ABC" protocol of emergency resuscitation. Maintaining airway patency is essential for oxygenation. Issues that can lead to airway obstruction in patients with impaired consciousness or bulbar dysfunction include vomit or inability to clear secretions and mechanical blockage of the pharynx by the tongue, or laryngeal edema. In the Neuro-ICU population, intubation is mandatory to protect the airway when treating patients with refractory intracranial pressure (ICP) crises or refractory status epilepticus with general anesthetics.

11.3.2 Lung

Respiratory failure, either hypercapnic or hypoxic, requires intubation for invasive mechanical ventilation. Signs of impending respiratory failure include increased work of breathing with use of accessory muscles, difficulty speaking in full sentences, rapid shallow breaths, and nasal flaring. Common causes of hypoxic respiratory failure include atelectasis, aspiration, pneumonia, pulmonary edema, and pulmonary embolism. Patients with neuromuscular disease such as Guillain-Barré syndrome (GBS) or myasthenia gravis may require elective intubation in anticipation of impending respiratory failure as part of the disease course. The "20–30–40 rule" (vital capacity < 20 mL/kg, negative inspiratory force < 30 cm H_2O, maximal expiratory force < 40 cm H_2O, respectively) is a commonly cited pulmonary function threshold for intubation in GBS. As with all critically ill patients, the bedside clinical assessment should take precedence over these generic cutoff values in intubation decisions.

11.3.3 Tissue

The mantra of the Neuro-ICU is to prevent secondary brain injury. Recent trials have shown a potential benefit in avoiding brain hypoxia (brain tissue oxygen tension < 20 mm Hg).[1] Intubation plays an integral part in optimizing oxygen consumption in patients with brain injury. Intubation and sedation should be considered for patients with Glasgow coma score (GCS) < 8 as this will decrease energy expenditure and lead to improved brain oxygenation. Additionally, patients with ICP crises may require intubation for hyperventilation purposes.

11.4 Contraindications (and Precautions)

Aside from a "Do Not Intubate" (DNI) order, there are no true contraindications to intubation. There are situations in which the technique of intubation needs to adjusted and extra precautions taken. Therefore, proper assessment for a difficult airway is recommended in nonemergent cases.

11.4.1 General Assessment for Difficult Airway

Presence of the following physical characteristics should prompt consideration for potential difficult airway. Depending on the practitioner's comfort and skill level, consider alternate routes of intubation such as awake intubation by direct or video laryngoscopy, nasotracheal intubation, and flexible fiber-optic intubation.

- Cervical spine: The presence of possible neck instability (i.e., trauma) or limited mobility (i.e., short neck, prior surgery, rheumatoid arthritis) will restrict the ability to adequately position the patient and obtain a good view of the airway
- Patients with excessive facial hair, facial trauma, absence of teeth, and active oral or nasal bleeding may make it difficult to achieve a proper face-mask seal for effective ventilation
- Patients with limited mouth opening (typically less than three finger breadths)
- Patients with large tongue (i.e., Down syndrome) and poor visualization of the pharynx; a high Mallampati score is associated with difficult intubation (▶ Fig. 11.3)
- A short thyromental distance, from the Adam's apple to the chin, of less than three finger breadths is associated with an anterior airway and poor visualization during laryngoscopy (▶ Fig. 11.4)

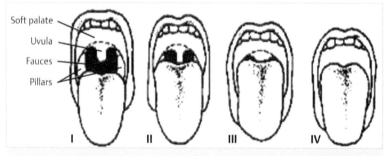

Fig. 11.3 Mallampati score.

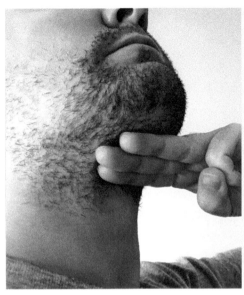

Fig. 11.4 Thyromental distance.

11.5 Equipment

Proper preparation is of utmost importance for successful intubation. It is essential to have all necessary equipment ready and easily accessible in anticipation of encountering a difficult airway. The mnemonic SOAP ME is useful as an initial equipment check[2]

- **S –** Suction turned on and ready to go
- **O –** Oxygen with bag-valve mask and nasal cannula @ 15 LPM
- **A –** Airway
  - Glidescope or laryngoscope (Mac or Miller blade)
  - Endotracheal tube (typically size 7 mm for adult women and 7.5–8.5 mm for adult men)
  - Stylet
  - Syringe (used to inflate cuff)
  - Oral airway, nasal airway
  - Supraglottic airway device (SAD)—laryngeal mask airway, esophageal-tracheal double-lumen airway
- **P –** Pharmacology (see ▶ Table 11.1)
  - Pretreat
  - Induction
  - Paralytic

Table 11.1 Pharmacological agents used for intubation

	Drug	Dose	Notes
Pretreat	Lidocaine	1–1.5 mg/kg	• Blunt hemodynamic and gag response to intubation ameliorating ICP elevations
Induction	Etomidate	0.1–0.3 mg/kg	• Raises blood pressure; caution in unsecured aneurysms or ICH • Transient adrenal suppression; not ideal for routine use in septic shock
	Ketamine	1–4 mg/kg	• Raises blood pressure and increases myocardial oxygen demand; caution in CAD, unsecured aneurysms, or ICH • Historically thought to increase ICP and CBV; however recent evidence has debunked this • Retains airway reflexes • Bronchodilator—useful for asthma
	Propofol	1–2 mg/kg	• Lowers blood pressure • Lowers ICP by decreasing cerebral metabolic rate for oxygen and thus decreases CBF and CBV in a hyperemic brain • Rapid onset, short acting • Provides amnesia; does not provide analgesia
	Midazolam	0.1–0.3 mg/kg	• Lowers blood pressure and ICP • Rapid onset, short acting • Provides amnesia; does not provide analgesia
Paralytic	Rocuro-nium	0.6–1 mg/kg	• Nondepolarizing agent • Rapid onset (1–2 min) • Lasts 60–90 min (longer in hepatic dysfunction)
	Cisatracur-ium	0.1–0.2 mg/kg	• Nondepolarizing agent • Slower onset (up to 5 min) • Last about 60 min, undergoes organ-independent elimination

	Succinylcho-line	1–1.5 mg/kg	• Depolari-zing agent; avoid in following:
			  ○ Neuromuscular disease
			  ○ Hyperkalemia
			  ○ Renal failure, burns, crush injuries
			  ○ Family history of malignant hyperthermia
			• Rapid onset (< 1 min)
			• Shortest duration (< 10 min)

Abbreviations: CAD, coronary artery disease; CBF, cerebral blood flow; CBV, cerebral blood volume; ICH, intracranial hemorrhage; ICP, intracranial pressure.

- **M** – Monitoring
  - SpO_2
  - Blood pressure
  - Electrocardiogram (ECG)
- **E** – End tidal CO_2

11.6 Technique

- Evaluate the patient for a potential difficult airway: As discussed in the preceding section, it is always best to have a backup plan if a difficult airway is anticipated.
- Pre-oxygenate/Ventilate: The ability to ventilate a patient is key and will bring ease of mind to the intubation team as this buys you time to wait for advanced backup to arrive (if needed). Inability to ventilate the patient is an emergency as this severely limits the time and number of intubation attempts before life-threatening hypoxia sets in.

In conscious patients, passive breathing of 100% oxygen for 5 minutes should provide adequate reserve for intubation. In unconscious patients, insertion of an oral or nasal airway is advised to help prevent the tongue from blocking air flow. Provide ventilation via face mask with good seal. Ensure good chest rise with appropriate oxygen saturation.

- Medicate: Once the patient is pre-oxygenated, proceed to pharmacological sedation followed by paralysis.

In patients with no cervical neck restriction, perform a head-tilt/chin-lift maneuver to place the head into a sniffing position (▶ Fig. 11.5). This helps

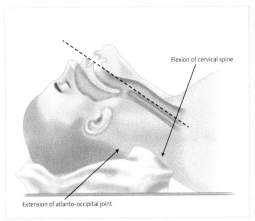

Fig. 11.5 Sniffing position.

Flexion of cervical spine

Extension of atlanto-occipital joint

prevent the tongue from obstructing the airway and aligns the airway for direct visualization.

11.6.1 Using Direct Laryngoscope (the Curved Macintosh Blade or the Straight Miller Blade)

- Scissor open the patient's mouth.
- Insert the blade in the right side of the patient's mouth and advance to the vallecula/base of tongue and sweep the tongue to the left (▶ Fig. 11.6).
- With the handle of the laryngoscope pointing away from you at 45 degrees, gently lift upwards and away. This will lift up the tongue and epiglottis and expose the vocal cords.
- The endotracheal tube is introduced and advanced through the vocal cords into the trachea.
- Once the endotracheal tube is advanced sufficiently, the stylet is removed.

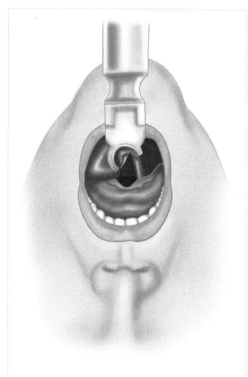

Fig. 11.6 Lateral displacement of tongue with direct laryngoscope.

11.6.2 Using Video Laryngoscope (Glidescope) —"Down, Up, Down, Up"

- Looking down at the patient's mouth, insert glidescope midline into the oral cavity until the tip of the scope is behind the tongue. No lateral tongue displacement is required.
- Looking up at the monitor, advance the glidescope until the epiglottis and vocal cords are visible. Anchor the tip of the glidescope into the vallecula.
- Looking down at the patient's mouth, insert the endotracheal tube into the oral cavity until the tube tip is near the distal tip of the glidescope. Try to avoid damaging the tonsils.
- Looking up at the monitor, advance the endotracheal tube through the vocal cords into the trachea while withdrawing the stylet.

Confirmation of Placement

The endotracheal tube is usually inserted to a distance of about three times the tube size (21 cm in a female with 7 mm endotracheal tube, 24 cm in a male with 8 mm endotracheal tube). Inflate the balloon and secure endotracheal tube. Confirm placement with a CO_2 detector, auscultation of bilateral breath sounds, and finally a chest X-ray.

11.6.3 Complications/Precautions

Complications that may occur during intubation include the following:
- Damaged to teeth, lips, and gums
- Damage to palate, tongue, tonsils, and vocal cords
- Malpositioned endotracheal tubes (esophagus vs. right main stem bronchus)
- Gastric distention and vomiting leading to aspiration
- Pneumothorax
- Hypoxia/hypercapnia in cases of difficult intubation

11.6.4 Difficult Airway Algorithm

It is essential to plan ahead for all intubations. Multiple professional organizations have published algorithms for unanticipated difficult airway. The 2015 Difficult Airway Society Algorithm[3] is shown in ▶ Fig. 11.7.

The algorithm essentially hinges on three levels: standard laryngoscopy → supraglottic assist devices (SAD) → surgical airway. If the patient is able to be easily ventilated using a SAD, then it is feasible to intubate via the SAD or perform a flexible fiber-optic intubation, depending on level of expertise available. Once the patient enters the "can't intubate, can't oxygenate" (CICO) situation, it is essential to have expert consultation to obtain a surgical airway (needle

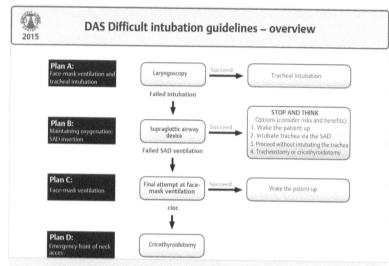

Fig. 11.7 Unanticipated difficult airway algorithm. (Reproduced from C. Frerk, V. S. Mitchell, A. F. McNarry, C. Mendonca, R. Bhagrath, A. Patel, E. P. O'Sullivan, N. M. Woodall and I. Ahmad, Difficult Airway Society 2015 guidelines for management of unanticipated difficult intubation in adults intubation guidelines working group. British Journal of Anaesthesia, 115 (6): 827–848 (2015).)

cricothyrotomy vs. surgical cricothyrotomy/tracheostomy vs. percutaneous tracheostomy).

11.6.5 Supraglottic Assist Devices

Laryngeal mask airway (LMA): The LMA is used as a temporizing measure to provide an airway and ventilation (when bag-valve mask ventilation is insufficient). To use, first deflate the cuff. Using index finger, press the device against the palate, with the face down, and insert until resistance is felt. Once situated in place, the cuff is inflated and a bag-valve mask is attached. Ensure breath sounds and chest rise with bagging see ▶ Fig. 11.8).

11.7 Expert Suggestions/Troubleshooting

- Rapid sequence intubation (RSI) is the simultaneous administration of sedative and paralytic. It is designed to help with rapid intubation and reduce aspiration risk, particularly in patients who have recently eaten. It is ideal for patients who do not have an examination suggestive of a difficult airway. Patients suspected of having a difficult airway should not undergo RSI (avoid

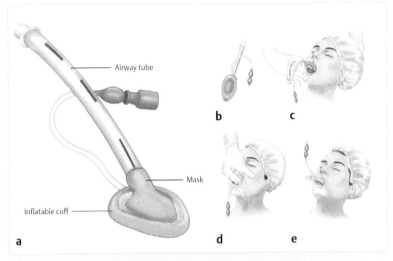

Fig. 11.8 (a-e) Laryngeal mask airway insertion technique.

paralytic). If paralytics are administered and the practitioner is unable to successfully intubate, then effective manual ventilation must be supplied until a more experienced practitioner arrives or the paralytic has worn off.

- Cricoid pressure was previously used routinely during RSI due to the belief that this downward force would help compress the esophagus and lower aspiration risk. New guidelines no longer recommend routine cricoid pressure as it does not reduce aspiration risk. It may however help improve visualization of the vocal cords during laryngoscopy.
- If a patient vomits during intubation, resist the urge to sit the patient up as this may drop the vomitus deeper into the airways. Instead, suction out what you can and proceed with intubation. Then place the patient in reverse Trendelenburg to facilitate suctioning any residual vomitus.
- One should be aware that positive pressure ventilation, after successful intubation, can cause hypotension especially in hypovolemic patients.
- Never be afraid to call for backup.

11.8 Special Circumstances

11.8.1 Intubation of Patients with Maxillofacial Injury

Maxillofacial trauma can cause airway obstruction, and may make intubation more difficult. Maxillofacial fractures may be classified as Le Fort type I, II, and

III fractures. Le Fort type I fractures occur horizontally below the inferior orbital rim, displacing the teeth and hard palate from the rest of the face. Le Fort type II fractures are triangular in shape and breach the inferior orbital rim, separating the maxilla from the zygoma and frontal bone. Le Fort type III fractures involve the orbital walls and zygomatic arch, allowing the facial bones to become separated from the face entirely. In all types of Le Fort fractures, the resulting edema and displacement of facial bones can obstruct the airway. Furthermore, Le Fort type II and III fractures can cause severe epistaxis and cerebrospinal fluid (CSF) leak, and may be associated with cervical spine and intracranial injury, further complicating airway management.

Emergent Situations

General principles to consider when managing the airway of patients with severe facial trauma:

- Bag-valve mask ventilation may not be possible due to bleeding or destruction of surrounding tissue, as this may prevent an appropriate seal between the mask and face. Use of supraglottic airway, such as LMA, may be considered.
- Both noninvasive ventilation and traditional intubation via direct laryngoscopy may be difficult due to blood or tissue disrupting the airway. In addition, the extent of facial injury or the co-existence of cervical spine injury requiring neck stabilization may reduce the extent to which the mouth and neck may be manipulated. Consider the use of video laryngoscopy, use of an elastic bougie, and/or fiber-optic bronchoscopy.
- When bleeding or tissue disruption are severe enough to make the above techniques prohibitively difficult, one may consider cricothyrotomy or tracheostomy.

Nonemergent Situations

General principles to consider when intubating a patient with facial trauma in the operating room:

- Assess the level of oral swelling, tongue swelling, airway edema, and tissue destruction. These may affect the extent to which the nose or mouth can be opened. This may be assessed both via physical examination and preoperative imaging.
- Consider whether or not nasal packing, throat packing, or fixation with hardware will be involved in the procedure.
- Based on the type of injury, nasal intubation may be considered as an alternative to orotracheal intubation.
- When skull base fractures are suspected, such as in Le Fort type II and III fractures, nasal intubation may be contraindicated. However, in certain

situations, nasal intubation is still used (especially if only small skull base fractures are suspected). Use of fiber-optic assistance is recommended when nasally intubating a patient with a suspected skull base fracture.

- If nasal intubation cannot be used for the procedure, submental intubation or tracheostomy may be performed. Note that submental intubation requires the patient to be initially orally intubated, after which point a tube is passed via a submental incision through the floor of the mouth. LMA tubes may also be used with this procedure.
- If both oral and nasal intubation cannot be used, consider tracheostomy.

11.8.2 Intubation of Patients with Cervical Spine Trauma[4,5]

When intubating a patient who has sustained injury to the cervical spine and requires cervical spine immobilization, it is important to take care to minimize c-spine manipulation. In a study using cadavers, it was found that bag-valve mask ventilation resulted in the most displacement of the cervical spine, while nasal intubation caused the least displacement (2.93 mm vs. 1.20 mm). Oral intubation caused 1.51 mm of displacement on average.[6] Thus, the neck must be immobilized during intubation in all patients suspected of c-spine injury until injury can be ruled out.

Typically, a cervical collar is used in patients requiring c-spine immobilization. However, it significantly impedes mouth opening necessary to place an endotracheal tube. Thus, manual inline stabilization is recommended during intubation. Manual inline stabilization consists of removal of the anterior aspect of the collar and manually stabilizing the patient's head and neck in neutral position, while resisting the forces applied to the neck during intubation. While this will make visualization of the vocal cords more difficult during laryngoscopy, it is recommended in order to maximize protection of the spine. In a cadaver study, it has been shown that manual inline stabilization is more effective than use of c-collar alone in decreasing c-spine subluxation.[7]

Principles to Consider

Using a gum-elastic bougie may facilitate intubation and assist in minimizing c-spine movement when the provider is unable to maximally open the mouth due to c-spine stabilization.

- Video laryngoscopy may be considered as an alternative to direct laryngoscopy, as it requires less opening of the mouth, and may thus be easier to perform when the c-spine is immobilized.
- Awake fiber-optic intubation carries the advantage of allowing one to perform a neurological examination before and after intubation (as opposed to intubation with rapid induction of anesthesia). Consider this method

when intubating patients with known or suspected unstable cervical injury in order to preserve neurological examination.

- LMA may be used as an alternative to traditional endotracheal tubes; however, this remains controversial as some authors report greater c-spine movement with use of LMA.

11.8.3 Intubation of Patients with Dislodged Tracheostomy Tube[8,9]

In the Neuro-ICU population, neurologically injured patients often require repeated intubation and subsequent long-term definitive airway placement. It is important to realize that if a recently placed tracheostomy tube (i.e., less than 2 weeks old) should become dislodged, reinsertion should be done with the utmost caution. Reinsertion can lead to a false passage being formed as the surgical tract may not be fully formed. Ventilation into a false passage leads to creation and expansion of subcutaneous emphysema, worsening of ventilation, and unanticipated difficult intubation. Ultimately, this may lead to eventual difficulty in securing the airway and possible death. It is better to reintubate the patient using either direct or video laryngoscopy.

11.8.4 Intubation of Patients Post Carotid Endarterectomy or Cervical Spine Surgery[10]

Postoperatively, after carotid endarterectomy or cervical spine surgery, neck hematoma formation risks loss of airway. Should expanding hematoma risk loss of airway, securing the airway should be done with the patient awake and with surgical assistance at the bedside capable of opening the sutures and releasing pressure from the hematoma.

11.8.5 Intubation of Patients Post Transphenoidal Surgery

Postoperatively, after transphenoidal surgery, it is important to be aware that bag-valve mask ventilation is relatively contraindicated. After breach of the sphenoid bone, air enters the cranium; thus, bag-valve mask ventilation expands the air and risks tension pneumocephalus. Ventilation should then be done through LMA.

11.8.6 Intubation of Patients with Moya-Moya

During induction in patients with Moya-Moya, one must keep blood pressure and pCO_2 elevated to avoid watershed ischemia. This is in contrast to cerebral edema and high ICP situations in which hyperemia is harmful and systolic blood pressure goals are typically aimed at less than 160.

11.8.7 Intubation of Morbidly Obese Patients

Caution should be taken when inducing general anesthesia on the following patients: morbidly obese patients, patients with sleep apnea, head and neck tumors, facial trauma, and/or facial burns. A difficult airway cart with fiber-optic scopes should be available and/or awake intubation selected as the initial technique. Morbidly obese patients should have a ramp to align the axis and optimize sniffing position.

References

[1] Okonkwo DO, Shutter LA, Moore C, et al. Brain oxygen optimization in severe traumatic brain injury phase-II: a phase II randomized trial. Crit Care Med. 2017; 45(11):1907–1914

[2] Back 2 Basics Series: Your Simple RSI Checklist - SOAP ME. 2014. https://em.umaryland.edu/educational_pearls/2577/. Accessed February 19, 2018

[3] Frerk C, Mitchell VS, McNarry AF, et al. Difficult Airway Society intubation guidelines working group. Difficult Airway Society 2015 guidelines for management of unanticipated difficult intubation in adults. Br J Anaesth. 2015; 115(6):827–848

[4] Austin N, Krishnamoorthy V, Dagal A. Airway management in cervical spine injury. Int J Crit Illn Inj Sci. 2014; 4(1):50–56

[5] Jung JY. Airway management of patients with traumatic brain injury/C-spine injury. Korean J Anesthesiol. 2015; 68(3):213–219

[6] Hauswald M, Sklar DP, Tandberg D, Garcia JF. Cervical spine movement during airway management: cinefluoroscopic appraisal in human cadavers. Am J Emerg Med. 1991; 9(6):535–538

[7] Gerling MC, Davis DP, Hamilton RS, et al. Effects of cervical spine immobilization technique and laryngoscope blade selection on an unstable cervical spine in a cadaver model of intubation. Ann Emerg Med. 2000; 36(4):293–300

[8] Lerner AD, Yarmus L. Percutaneous dilational tracheostomy. Clin Chest Med. 2018; 39(1):211–222

[9] Morris LL, Whitmer A, McIntosh E. Tracheostomy care and complications in the intensive care unit. Crit Care Nurse. 2013; 33(5):18–30

[10] Shakespeare WA, Lanier WL, Perkins WJ, Pasternak JJ. Airway management in patients who develop neck hematomas after carotid endarterectomy. Anesth Analg. 2010; 110(2):588–593

12 Cricothyrotomy

David F. Slottje, Adam D. Fox, and Matthew Vibbert

Abstract

Cricothyrotomy (aka cricothyroidotomy) is an emergent procedure, performed in order to establish an airway in a patient with respiratory failure who cannot be oxygenated and ventilated via alternative measures. Here the following topics related to cricothyrotomy are discussed in detail: relevant anatomy and physiology, indications/contraindications, equipment, technique, complications, and expert suggestions.

Keywords: cricothyrotomy, tracheostomy, respiratory failure, intubation, surgical airway

12.1 Introduction

A cricothyrotomy is a temporary surgical airway, created by incising the anterior neck in the midline and inserting an endotracheal or tracheostomy tube through the cricothyroid membrane into the trachea. It is performed in the emergent setting of life-threatening respiratory compromise in a patient who can be neither intubated nor ventilated via alternative measures.

12.2 Relevant Anatomy and Physiology

Successful cricothyrotomy relies on a basic knowledge of the surface anatomy of the anterior neck and the underlying laryngeal structures. In the midline, several important landmarks are usually palpable. The hyoid bone can be felt as a hard but mobile arch just below the angle of the chin. The thyroid notch can be felt two finger-breadths below the hyoid bone, as a firm V-shaped depression. The thyroid notch is the superior border of the thyroid cartilage which continues inferiorly at a distance of approximately two finger-breadths. The two halves of the thyroid cartilage can be felt extending laterally. The cricoid cartilage is the next rigid structure, palpated immediately below the thyroid cartilage. There is a soft declivity between the thyroid and cricoid cartilages spanning less than one finger-breadth. This is the cricothyroid membrane through which a cricothyrotomy is created. The tracheal rings and overlying thyroid gland are palpable inferior to the cricoid cartilage. The sternal notch lies at the base of the neck (see ▸ Fig. 12.1 and ▸ Fig. 12.2).

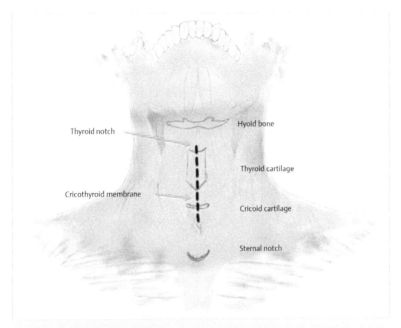

Fig. 12.1 Neck surface landmarks.

The only intervening tissue layers between the skin surface and the cricothyroid membrane are the epidermis, dermis, superficial cervical fascia containing subcutaneous adipose tissue, and the investing and pretracheal layers of the deep cervical fascia. Practically, these tissue layers are quite thin (with the exception of subcutaneous adipose tissue which may be variable). To the naked eye, the layers will appear as a skin, a variable amount of fat, and a veil of fascia overlying the cricothyroid membrane (see ▶ Fig. 12.3). Platysma and strap muscles (sternohyoid, omohyoid, thyrohyoid, and sternothyroid) are typically absent in the midline at the level of the cricoid cartilage (see ▶ Fig. 12.4 and ▶ Fig. 12.5). The innominate artery crosses the lower trachea from left to right and is typically well below the site of cricothyrotomy.

Identification of the cricothyroid membrane by palpation may be difficult or impossible in the setting of obesity, a short and stout neck, neck trauma, neck mass, or prior neck surgery. In such circumstances a large incision may be necessary to successfully perform a cricothyrotomy.

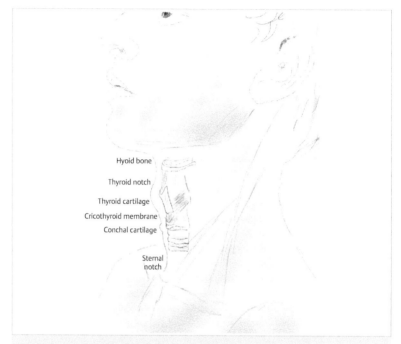

Hyoid bone
Thyroid notch
Thyroid cartilage
Cricothyroid membrane
Conchal cartilage

Sternal
notch

Fig. 12.2 Lateral profile of neck surface anatomy.

12.3 Indications

Cricothyrotomy is indicated for a patient in respiratory failure who cannot be intubated or ventilated. Alternative procedures include fiber-optic intubation, insertion of a supraglottic airway device, retrograde intubation, needle cricothyrotomy, and tracheostomy. (The approach to a difficult airway is reviewed in detail in Chapter 11, Intubation.) Ultimately, cricothyrotomy is the rescue procedure of choice when such alternative procedures have been attempted without success or when the patient is in extremis. Specific clinical scenarios which may require cricothyrotomy are multifarious and include upper airway obstruction/inflammation, oral/facial trauma, airway hemorrhage, neck trauma/hematoma, oropharyngeal or neck mass, and congenital deformities.

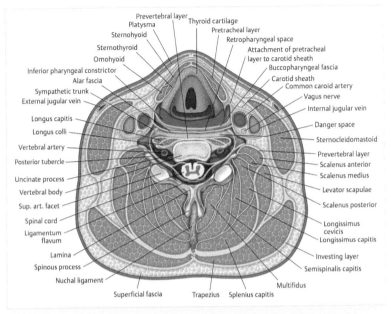

Fig. 12.3 Transverse section of neck at the level of C5 (Reproduced from Subaxial Cervical Spine. In: Vialle L, Hrsg. AOSpine Masters Series, Volume 5: Cervical Spine Trauma. 1st ed. Thieme; 2015.)

12.4 Contraindications

There are no absolute contraindications to cricothyrotomy but alternative surgical airways are preferred in certain scenarios. When there is suspected transection of the larynx or upper trachea, a tracheostomy should be performed to establish the airway below the level of injury. In patients under the age of 12 cricothyrotomy carries an increased risk of permanent laryngeal injury.[1] As such, needle cricothyrotomy or tracheostomy is usually performed in the pediatric population.

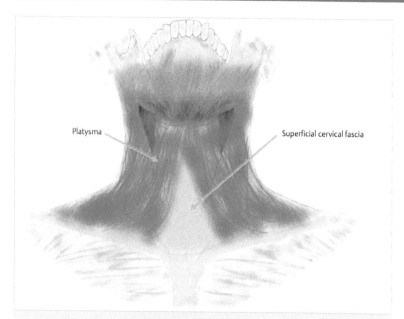

Fig. 12.4 Subcutaneous structures of neck.

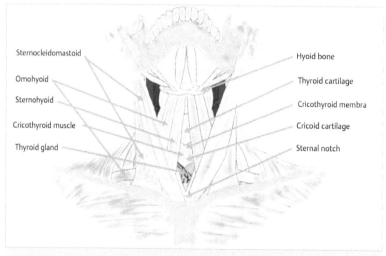

Fig. 12.5 Subfascial structures of neck.

12.5 Equipment

If required, cricothyrotomy can be performed using only a scalpel and an endotracheal tube, tracheostomy tube, or other canula. In general, the procedure should not be delayed to gather additional supplies. When time and availability permit, the following equipment may be helpful:

- Cap, mask, gown, sterile gloves, perforated sterile drape
- Marking pen
- Gauze
- Chlorhexidine gluconate or betadine skin prep
- Light source
- Suction
- #15 or #10 blade scalpel
- Mosquito clamp or tracheal spreader
- Electrocautery
- Self-retaining retractor
- Tracheal hook
- Bougie
- 6.0 endotracheal tube (flexible tipped tube preferred) or 6.0 tracheostomy tube
- Stylet
- 10 cc syringe
- Ambu bag
- Oxygen source
- End tidal CO_2 detector
- 2–0 silk sutures

12.6 Technique

12.6.1 Preparation

- A team effort should be made with all available personnel to gather the aforementioned equipment.
- In addition to the primary operator, an assistant familiar with performing cricothyrotomy can be extremely helpful.

12.6.2 Medications

- An attempt should be made to ventilate the patient and deliver 100% oxygen. Oxygen content should be turned down if it becomes necessary to utilize electrocautery in or around the airway.
- Antibiotics are not necessary.

- Usually, patients requiring cricothyrotomy are obtunded. If necessary, sedation can be accomplished with etomidate, propofol, midazolam, ketamine and/or fentanyl. In a hypotensive patient, etomidate is the agent of choice.
- Lidocaine with epinephrine can be used for local anesthesia if time permits.

12.6.3 Positioning/Equipment Set-up

- Position the patient supine with a shoulder roll placed horizontally behind the scapula and the neck extended (unless contraindicated).
- If there is time, mark out the thyroid notch, cricoid cartilage, sternal notch, and a 5 cm vertical incision in the midline centered over the cricothyroid membrane.
- Train any available lights on the surgical site.
- Don a sterile gown, cap, facemask, and gloves.
- Apply sterile prep and drape the neck.
- Inject local anesthetic at the incision site in an awake patient.
- A right-handed physician should stand on the patient's right side to perform the procedure and a left-handed physician should stand on the left.

12.6.4 Procedure

- Pinch the thyroid cartilage with the nondominant hand to assist with orientation and stabilize the larynx.
- Make a generous midline vertical incision centered over the cricothyroid membrane. This should be extended if needed.
- Divide the subcutaneous tissue and superficial fascia. (In reality, the incision can often be made straight down to the cricothyroid membrane.)
- Place a self-retaining retractor into the wound if one is available.
- Palpate the cricoid cartilage.
- Spread the deep cervical fascia with the mosquito clamp, exposing the cricothyroid membrane.
- Incise the cricothyroid membrane horizontally with the knife.
- Advance the mosquito clamp into the airway. (A tracheal hook can also be used at this point.)
- Spread the clamp to widen the opening in the cricothyroid membrane. (If no clamp is available, the blunt end of the scalpel can be inserted into the airway and twisted to accomplish the same purpose.)
- Once the cricothyrotomy has been performed the airway should be secured using an available tracheostomy or endotracheal tube. A bougie can be used to maintain access to the airway if readily available.
- Remove the stylet if one is used.
- Inflate the endotracheal or tracheostomy tube cuff.

- Connect the endotracheal or tracheostomy tube to an ambu bag or ventilator.
- Confirm appropriate return of end-tidal CO_2.
- An assistant should auscultate to confirm bilateral breath sounds.
- Assess adequacy of oxygen delivery.
- Achieve hemostasis.
- If an endotracheal tube is used, it can be secured with two "Roman Sandal" 2–0 silk sutures and tape. A tracheostomy tube can be directly sutured to the neck with 2–0 silk sutures.
- Dress the wound with gauze.
- Obtain a chest X-ray to confirm appropriate placement and to rule out pneumothorax.

See ▶ Fig. 12.6, ▶ Fig. 12.7, ▶ Fig. 12.8, ▶ Fig. 12.9, and ▶ Fig. 12.10.

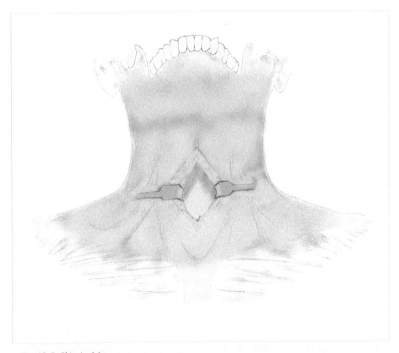

Fig. 12.6 Skin incision.

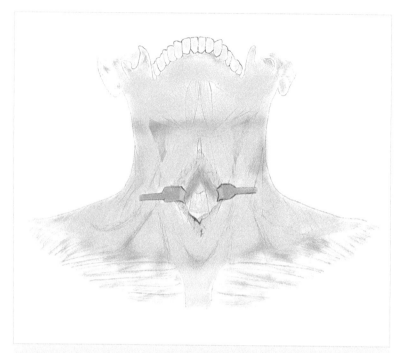

Fig. 12.7 Exposure of deep cervical fascia.

12.7 Complications

Emergent cricothyrotomy carries a 15% risk of complication.[2]

12.7.1 Acute Complications

- Bleeding
  - Small veins overlying the cricothyroid membrane can cause significant bleeding and should be coagulated, if necessary, once the airway is established.
  - Innominate artery injury is possible but much less likely than with tracheostomy.
- Pneumothorax
  - This may occur from the cricothyrotomy itself or from aggressive attempts to bag-valve ventilate during the procedure.
- Esophageal injury

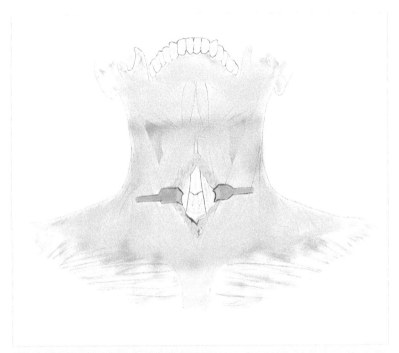

Fig. 12.8 Exposure of cricothyroid membrane.

- Vocal cord injury
- Injury to adjacent neurovascular structures
- Subcutaneous emphysema
  - Occurs with misplacement or dislodgement of the endotracheal tube.

12.7.2 Delayed Complications

- Subglottic stenosis
  - Traditionally, it has been believed that a cricothyrotomy should be converted to a tracheostomy within 72 hours to mitigate risk of subglottic stenosis,[3] although there is some evidence to suggest that this may be unnecessary.
  - In some cases, the cricoid cartilage may need to be repaired. In this situation an ear, nose, and throat (ENT) surgeon should be consulted to assist with revision of the cricothyrotomy to tracheostomy.
- Infection

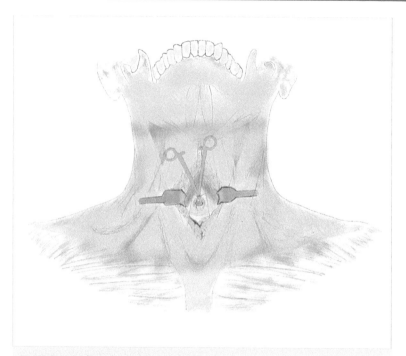

Fig. 12.9 Spreading of cricothyroid membrane.

- Tracheal-innominate fistula
  - This deadly complication is much less common with cricothyrotomy than with tracheostomy given the inferior location of the innominate artery. It is believed to result from chronic infection of the surgical site or tracheal necrosis from cuff hyperinflation. It will usually present in 3 to 4 weeks following insertion of the surgical airway with massive hemoptysis. In some cases, this is preceded by "sentinel bleeding." Pulsation of the airway with the heartbeat is a helpful diagnostic clue. The first step in management is to hyperinflate the airway cuff. If this does not stop the bleeding and if the ostomy tract is mature (> 7–10 days old), the airway should be removed and an endotracheal tube should be passed through the ostomy. If the ostomy is not mature, oral endotracheal intubation should be performed and the surgical airway should be removed once the endotracheal tube is through vocal cords. Once an airway is established and the lungs are protected from hemorrhage, the patient should be transported to the operating room for sternotomy and surgical repair of the fistula. Several maneuvers have been described to temporize bleeding in the interim.

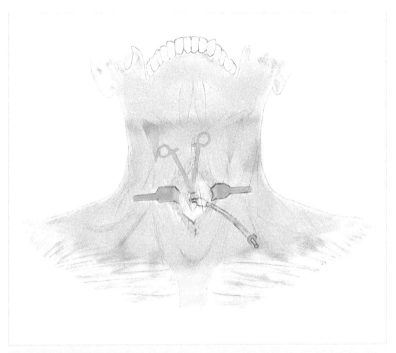

Fig. 12.10 Insertion of endotracheal tube.

- If a tracheostomy tube is still in place, it can be torqued upward to apply pressure to the innominate artery.
- The "Little Dutch Boy Maneuver" entails placing a finger through the ostomy site, dissecting the soft tissue bluntly to the level of sternum, and compressing the innominate artery against inner wall of the sternal notch (see ▶ Fig. 12.11).
- The "Utley Maneuver" is performed by making a right infraclavicular incision, through which a finger is inserted to compress the innominate artery.

12.8 Expert Suggestions/Troubleshooting

12.8.1 Controlled Chaos

Inherently, cricothyrotomy is a highly emergent procedure with life or death implications for the patient. Accordingly, it is incumbent upon the physician

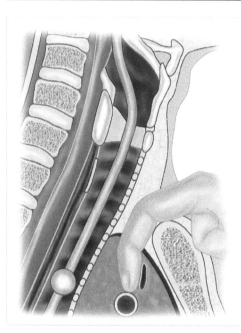

Fig. 12.11 Little Dutch Boy Maneuver.

performing the procedure to provide calm leadership. A coordinated and efficient team effort, utilizing all available personnel, will maximize the odds of a favorable patient outcome.

12.8.2 Time Management

The acuity of a specific clinical situation may mandate skipping many of the aforementioned procedural steps. There are some steps, however, that will ultimately save time and should not be skipped. These include extending the neck (if able), illuminating the surgical field (a cell phone light can be used if no other light source is available), making a large enough incision, and properly identifying the site of the cricothyroid membrane.

12.8.3 Don't Lose the Airway

Once the airway is entered, an instrument or finger should maintain constant contact with the opening until the endotracheal tube or a bougie is inserted.

References

[1] Patel SA, Meyer TK. Surgical airway. Int J Crit Illn Inj Sci. 2014; 4(1):71–76

[2] Smith MD, Katrinchak J. Use of a gum elastic bougie during surgical crichothyrotomy. Am J Emerg Med. 2008; 26(6):738.e1

[3] Talving P, DuBose J, Inaba K,. Demetriades D.. Conversion of emergent cricothyrotomy to tracheostomy in trauma patients. Arch Surg. 2010; 145(1):87–91

13 Chest Tube Insertion

Amna Sheikh and Amandeep S. Dolla

Abstract

Chest tubes are plastic tubes inserted into the pleural cavity for drainage of fluid or air. This chapter will explain the indications, contraindications, techniques, and complications of the procedure. Both standard and Seldinger techniques for insertion are described.

Keywords: chest tube, pneumothorax, hemothorax, empyema, pleural effusion

13.1 Introduction

A chest tube is a sterile silicone or polyvinyl chloride (PVC) tube inserted into the pleural cavity through the chest wall for drainage of fluid (pleural effusion, empyema, hemothorax) or air (pneumothorax). It is usually done as a bedside procedure but sometimes is performed in the operating room (OR) after thoracic surgery.

13.2 Relevant Anatomy/Physiology

The space between the lung and chest wall is called the pleural space. It is lined by a single layer of mesothelium called pleura. Parietal pleura supplied by intercostal vessels covers the chest wall and visceral pleura supplied by pulmonary vessels lines the lung. An extensive lymphatic network that drains into the thoracic duct lines both pleural surfaces.

Parietal capillaries, visceral capillaries, and interstitium generate the pleural fluid. Visceral capillaries have lower pressure than the parietal capillaries. The summation of hydrostatic and oncotic pressure gradients between the pleural and plasma facilitates the production of pleural fluid. Pleural fluid is drained by lymphatics and capillaries at an estimated rate of 20 mL/hour/hemithorax[1] in a 70 kg man.

13.3 Indications

13.3.1 Emergency Indications

- Pneumothorax: Pneumothorax is defined as entry of air in the pleural space. It can be traumatic, iatrogenic, or spontaneous. Treatment involves removing air from the space, helping the lung to re-expand and to prevent re-accumulation of air. Chest tubes are indicated in pneumothorax patients if they are clinically unstable, are on mechanical ventilation, or exhibit signs of tension pneumothorax, or if the pneumothorax is large or occurs as a result of trauma.

- Hemothorax: Management for hemothorax includes resuscitation and drainage to ensure lung inflation and monitoring for blood loss. Complete drainage of blood is important to prevent empyema and fibrothorax.[2]
- Esophageal rupture with gastric leak into pleural space. Chest tube is placed mostly postoperatively in these patients.

13.3.2 Nonemergent Indications

- Pleural effusions: Accumulation of fluid in the pleural space could be either transudative or exudative based on the composition of the fluid and etiology. Para-pneumonic and large recurrent transudative pleural effusions require chest tubes for drainage.
- Empyema: Drainage of empyema is required for source control.
- Chylothorax.
- Treatment with sclerosing agents or pleurodesis.
- Postoperative care.

13.4 Contraindications

- No absolute contraindications to the procedure.
- Coagulopathy: If the patient is on anticoagulants or has a bleeding disorder there is a risk of bleeding with the procedure.[3] Assess the risks versus benefits before proceeding. If a chest tube needs to be placed emergently, simultaneous correction of the bleeding disorder should be carried out.
- Hepatohydrothorax: Cirrhotic patients with transudative effusions should not be managed with chest tubes.[3]
- Pulmonary blebs.
- Complete adhesion of the lung to chest wall.

13.5 Equipment

Chest tube kits usually come with all the required materials (▶ Fig. 13.1). Below is a list of materials needed:
- Sterile gown and gloves
- Chlorhexidine
- Sterile drape
- 1% lidocaine
- 10-mL syringe and a 20-mL syringe

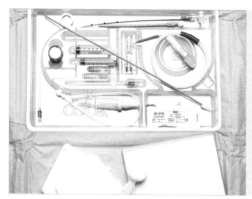

Fig. 13.1 Chest tube kit. Courtesy: Cook Medical.

Table 13.1 Size of chest tubes

Indication	Size	Technique
Tension pneumothorax	14–28	Needle decompression then Seldinger
Pleural effusion (Transudate or malignancy)	14–16	Seldinger
Empyema	16–28	Seldinger-Standard
Hemothorax	18–40	Seldinger-Standard
Parapneumonic	14–24	Seldinger
Bronchopleural fistula	20–28	Seldinger-Standard

- One small-gauge needle (size 25) and one large-gauge needle for deeper anesthetic infiltration (size 18–21)
- Several dissecting instruments, such as curved Kelly clamps or hemostats
- Needle driver
- Scissors
- 0 silk sutures
- Chest tube of appropriate size (see ▶ Table 13.1).
- Pleural drainage system, such as the Pleur-evac (Teleflex Medical), should also be ready for connection after the chest tube is inserted.

13.6 Technique

13.6.1 Preparation

- Positioning: Place the patient in a supine or semi-recumbent position. Place the ipsilateral arm behind the patient's head.

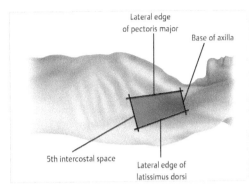

Fig. 13.2 Triangle of safety.

Lateral edge
of pectoris major

Base of axilla

5th intercostal space

Lateral edge of
latissimus dorsi

- Site: Chest tubes placed emergently (without image guidance) should enter the thorax through the "triangle of safety" (▶ Fig. 13.2). This safe zone is defined by the anterior border of latissimus dorsi, the lateral border of pectoralis major, and a horizontal line at the level of the nipple (in males) or the infra-mammillary crease (in females)—both of which correspond approximately to the fourth intercostal space. The apex of the triangle lies just below the axilla. In nonemergent scenarios in which ultrasound guidance is utilized, it may be desirable to enter through a lower intercostal space (e.g., as low as possible for pleural effusion).
- After identifying the spot for insertion, mark it with a pen.
- Procedure should be performed under full barrier precautions.
- Clean the area with chlorhexidine and drape the patient to create a large sterile field, with only the marked area exposed.
- Anesthetize the area with 1 to 2% lidocaine. Make sure to anesthetize the skin, subcutaneous tissue, chest wall muscles, rib periosteum, and the pleura. Use your finger to guide the needle on top of the rib. Keeping negative pressure, advance the needle until flash of pleural fluid in case of effusion or air in case of pneumothorax enters the syringe. Inject the remaining lidocaine to anesthetize the pleura.
- Withdraw the needle and the syringe completely.
- In cases of penetrating chest trauma, a single dose of prophylactic antibiotics should be administered prior to the procedure.

13.6.2 Seldinger Technique (▶ Fig. 13.3)

- Once the area has been anesthetized insert the introducer needle while maintaining negative pressure.
- Once fluid or air is aspirated, pass the guidewire through the needle.
- Remove the needle and create a small stab incision in the skin at the entry site.

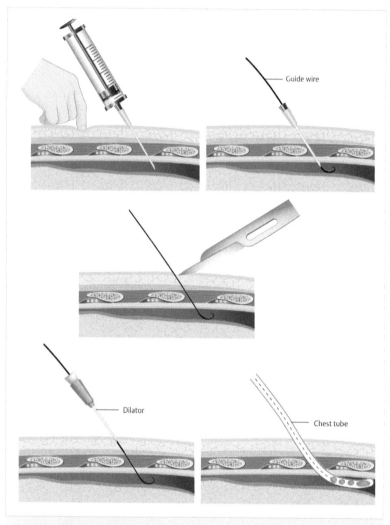

Fig. 13.3 Seldinger technique.

- Pass the dilators sequentially over the guidewire.
- Once the area is dilated, pass the chest tube over the guidewire such that all of the drainage holes are completely within the pleural space, and then remove the guidewire.
- Attach a three-way stopcock to the chest tube.

- Secure the chest tube in place by a 0 silk purse string suture.
- Connect the chest tube to an underwater seal with negative pressure.
- Confirm placement with a chest X-ray.

13.6.3 Standard Technique (▶ Fig. 13.4)

- Position and prepare the patient for the procedure as described above.
- After anesthetizing the area with lidocaine, make a 2 to 3 cm long transverse incision over the center of the rib.
- Take a Kelly clamp or hemostat and dissect through the subcutaneous tissue until you reach the rib surface.
- Pass the instrument along the superior border of the rib and dissect through the intercostal fascia and muscle into the parietal pleura.
- Insert a finger in the pleural space to avoid any adjacent lung injury and clear the area of any debris. Remove the Kelly clamp.
- Mount the chest tube onto the Kelly clamp and insert it alongside finger into the pleural cavity, ensuring that all drainage holes are completely within the pleural space. Direct the tube anterosuperiorly for pneumothorax and posteroinferiorly for fluid.
- Secure the chest tube in place with 0 silk purse string sutures. Apply a sterile dressing on top. Petroleum dressing is not necessary.
- Connect the chest tube with a collection system on low wall suction.

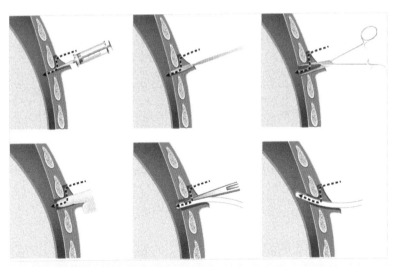

Fig. 13.4 Standard technique.

- Confirm placement with chest X-ray by following the radio-opaque line on the tube.
- If the proximal drainage hole is outside the pleural space, the tube will need to be replaced.

13.7 Removal

Determination of when to remove a chest tube varies based upon indication.
- Pleural effusion: Criteria for removal
  - Patient shows clinical improvement
  - The volume is < 200 mL in 24 hours[4]
  - Fluid is serous[4]
  - Lung has re-expanded on chest X-ray
- Pneumothorax: Criteria for removal
  - Initially chest tube is placed to wall suction.
  - Once the lung has fully expanded it can be placed to water seal.
  - Once there is no air leak present, the chest tube can be clamped.
  - If there is no air leak and no re-accumulation of pneumothorax on chest X-ray, after 12 to 24 hours the chest tube can be removed.

13.7.1 Technique for Removal

Two personnel should be involved in removing chest tubes.

Mechanically Ventilated Patient

Decision to remove the tube should be made cautiously in high risk mechanically ventilated patients such as those requiring high FiO₂, with high positive end-expiratory pressure (PEEP), with history of recurrent pneumothorax, and with history of chronic lung disease. Once the decision has been made to remove the tube the following procedure should be followed[4]
- Tube should be removed during end-expiration.
- Cut the sutures and pull the tube quickly.
- Quickly occlude the site with gauze.
- If needed, place extra sutures at the entry site although it will usually close and heal best by secondary intention.
- Apply pressure dressing. Petroleum dressing is not necessary.
- Chest radiograph should be obtained 12 to 24 hours after removal.[4]

Spontaneously Breathing Patient

- Ask the patient to do a Valsalva maneuver or to inhale deeply after full exhalation, and then the tube should be removed.
- Rest of the procedure is the same as in a mechanically ventilated patient.

13.8 Complications

- Pain: It is a common complication in patients with chest tube. Pain should be adequately managed.
- Bleeding: It occurs mostly due to injury to intercostal vessels.
- Infection: In traumatic hemothorax, the incidence of empyema ranges from 0 to 18%.[5] In cases of penetrating chest trauma, use of a single dose of prophylactic antibiotics at the time of chest tube insertion decreases the incidence of infection.[6] There is no data to support use of prophylactic antibiotics in patients with blunt injuries or nontraumatic indications for chest tube placement.
- Lung laceration: It occurs with trocars or clamps. A sudden thrust into the chest cavity can cause damage to the lung, nerves, vessels, and solid organs.
- Mediastinal injury.
- Solid organ puncture.
- Intercostal vessels and nerve laceration.
- Re-expansion of pulmonary edema: It is rare but potentially fatal complication. It can occur immediately or within 24 hours. Patients develop tachycardia, tachypnea, and hypoxia. Treatment includes oxygenation, diuresis if tolerated, hemodynamic support and low threshold for mechanical ventilation.[2]
- Long thoracic nerve laceration.

13.9 Expert Suggestions/Troubleshooting

- Chest tubes in patients with positive pressure ventilation should be assessed often.
- If a moderate or a severe air leak stops suddenly, the chest tube should be checked for blockages or kinking.[2] Blockages can sometimes be cleared by stripping the drainage tubing. When this is unsuccessful, the chest tube can also be rotated by 360 degrees and/or pulled back 1 to 2 cm if there is sufficient length of tubing within the pleural space. The tube can also be sterilely disconnected and suctioned with a flexible endotracheal suction cannula or mechanically cleared with a Fogarty balloon.
- In patients with a history of prior pulmonary surgery or pleurodesis, it may be preferable to place a chest tube under ultrasound or computed tomography (CT) guidance.
- In the case of malposition of a chest tube within the lung parenchyma, a second chest tube must be placed in the pleural space prior to removal of the malpositioned tube in anticipation of significant bleeding and/or air leak.

References

[1] Broaddus VC, Wiener-Kronish JP, Berthiaume Y, Staub NC. Removal of pleural liquid and protein by lymphatics in awake sheep. J Appl Physiol (1985). 1988; 64(1):384–390

[2] Dev SP, Nascimiento B, Jr, Simone C, Chien V. Videos in clinical medicine: chest-tube insertion. N Engl J Med. 2007; 357(15):e15

[3] Lotano VE. Chest tube thoracostomy. In: Parrillo JE DR, ed. Critical Care Medicine: Principles of Diagnosis and Management in the Adult. Elsevier, Saunders; 2014

[4] Arya R, Rajaram SS. Chest tube (tube thoracostomy) placement. In: Rajaram S, ed. Critical Care Procedure Book. Nova Science Publishers, Inc; 2015

[5] Olivas VJ. Chest tube placement. In: Kupesic Plavsic P, ed. Urgent Procedures in Medical Practice. New Delhi: Jaypee Brothers Medical Publishers Ltd; 2017:95–99

[6] Luchette FA, Barrie PS, Oswanski MF, et al. Eastern Association for Trauma. Practice management guidelines for prophylactic antibiotic use in tube thoracostomy for traumatic hemopneumothorax: the EAST Practice Management Guidelines Work Group. J Trauma. 2000; 48(4):753–757

Index

Note: Page numbers set **bold** or *italic* indicate headings or figures, respectively.

151

Index

Index